Gastric Sleeve Bariatric Cookbook And Meal Plan

Easy, Tasty And Healthy Recipes For Every Stage Of Weight Loss Surgery, Before And After

AMY ZACKARY

DEDICATION

My Father in heaven,

Thank you!

TABLE OF CONTENTS

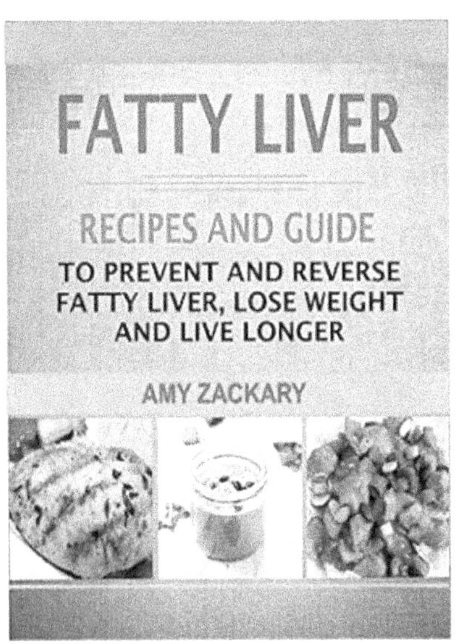

Fatty Liver: Recipes And Guide To Prevent And Reverse Fatty Liver, Lose Weight And Live Longer

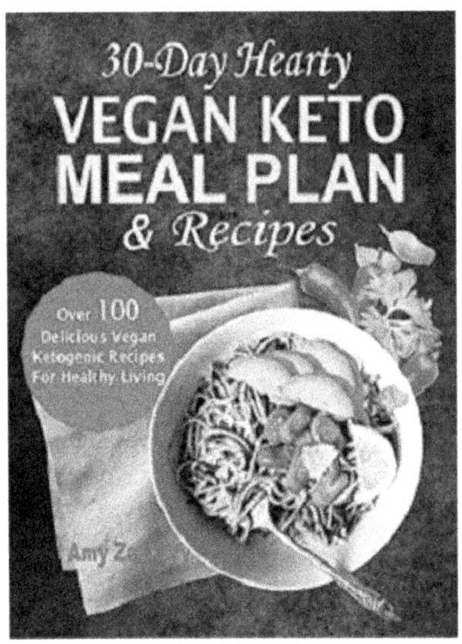

30-Day Hearty Vegan Keto Meal Plan & Recipes: Over 100 Delicious Vegan Ketogenic Recipes For Healthy Living

INTRODUCTION

Undergoing bariatric surgery takes effort, time, and money—but it works! This is why many people who are obese are finding succor in the permanency and effectiveness of this weight loss tool. It is a big deal; anyone who successfully goes through one deserves a huge congratulations. Their determination to lead a healthier and more productive life is laudable. That said, bariatric gastric surgery requires making some major lifestyle changes. Right from the moment you make a decision to undergo one, to living life after; you have to be sure of what to eat, when to eat it and how much of it to eat, before your surgery, and even after.

You see, it isn't just about taking off the excess weight alone; but following up on a strict eating regimen. Failure to do this will slow done recovery, or even worse, trigger other health issues. Even if your stomach has been altered to accommodate smaller amount of food, chronic overeating will gradually stretch the stomach to take in larger amounts of foods than originally intended. Thankfully, you have this book to guide you in a straightforward and simple way. For once you are in tuned with the right foods that your body needs, you can be sure of continual weight loss and ultimately, a sustained healthy weight.

So I want to congratulate for deciding to take the giant step to achieving a permanent healthier lifestyle. You deserve a healthier body and mind, and to really feel good about yourself. It is a wonderful experience and a life-changing one, and should be approached with all studiousness. If you follow the simple guidelines, meal plan and recipes that this book presents, you will be surprised at how easy it is at making this happen. Welcome to a life-changing and enjoyable gastric bypass experience!

Now, let's get to it!

Gastric Bypass Surgery And Your Diet

In a gastrostomy sleeve surgery, about 60 to 85% of the stomach is cut away. The stomach becomes small and takes the shape of a tube; just like a banana. The stomach's capacity to hold food and water in significantly lessened. Instead of holding its regular capacity of 3 pounds or 48 ounces of food, or even more in unusual circumstances, a sleeved stomach can now hold 10- 15 ounces of food. It becomes a small stomach that's neither flexible nor distensible.

A gastric diet is for people who are recovering from gastric bypass surgery (Roux-en-Y gastric bypass) and from sleeve gastrostomy. The diet helps them heal faster and to change the way they eat. Chewing the food is the first step, towards digestion, and the only conscious action a person takes towards it. You have to use your teeth to chew your foods and break them into small chunks before is passed down to the stomach through the esophagus. A smaller stomach of a gastric sleeve does not require large chunks of food. Once the food is swallowed, every other action becomes automatic.

So from the moment that you decide to go for a gastric bypass surgery, you have set yourself to embrace a life of change. Gastric sleeve surgery ensures that you eat only what your body needs. Nothing more! You can no longer eat whenever you feel like. You will have a different outlook to food and to look at it a whole new way.

It is therefore essential to create new habits and stop old ones that can increase weight and lead to obesity. Such habits include tracking your food intake in a food journal or in an online dairy, counting calories so as not to overeat, and participating in bariatric support group and establishing fitness goals. You will have to work closely with your professional healthcare provider, friends and relatives to build and maintain good habits from day to day.

Pre-Op Gastric Bypass Surgery Diet

Before your operation, it is important to follow a strict diet in order to reduce the size of your liver and minimize the risk of complications. This diet is known as the pre-operative diet and last for 2 to 3 weeks.

The liver is a large organ close to the stomach. Obesity enlarges the already large liver by storing excess glycogen, water and fatty deposits. An enlarged liver will make the operation more difficult. The pre-op diet will reduce these excess nutrients and reduce the size of the liver so that during operation, the liver can easily and safely be moved aside for easy access to the stomach. Your doctor may also ask you to lose some weight during this period. For many people, following a pre-op diet enables them to lose 5-10 pounds.

We eat plenty of carbs every day. We also take in lots of unhealthy fats. The pre-op diet will cut down on carbs and unhealthy fats. Foods like sweet potatoes, and pasta must be completely eliminated from your diet. Your pre-op diet should consist of lean proteins, vegetables and no-calorie fluids.

You will also need to drink at least 8- 12 ounces of liquids between meals, totaling 64 ounces per day. Drink at least 2 liters of fluid each day. Drink more when the weather is hot. Eliminate fluids like sodas, sweet tea, lattes and fruit juices completely from your diet. Avoid alcohol, caffeine and carbonated drinks. Eat and drink evenly throughout the day. This is a strict, calorie- reducing diet so stick to the daily calorie goal your doctor recommends for you.

2 days before the operation, your diet will consist of mostly clear liquid. This includes water, broth, decaffeinated coffee, sugar-free popsicles and

also one protein shake daily. Avoid carbonated beverages and caffeinated drinks.

You need lots of protein. The pre-op liquid diet puts the body into ketosis. This makes it possible for your body to burn the stored fat in your body and makes it its main energy source. Taking lots of protein- enriched drinks facilitates ketosis which shrinks the liver in a short time.

Your doctor may also recommend that you take daily bariatric supplements to supply your body with the required nutrient before operation.

It will be helpful if you count your calories before you eat. This is a good habit to develop and will help you even after surgery. Remain hydrated all through this period. Do not eat any solid food while you are on the all liquid diet. The liquids must be low in calories and all soft drinks be completely ruled out.

On the midnight of the day scheduled for your surgery, do not take anything at all, liquid or solid. This is very important so that doctors can work on the stomach without interference from food or drinks. Failure to do this may cause complications or even death.

Post-Op Gastric Bypass Surgery Diet

The post- operation diet begins immediately after your surgery is completed. Your stomach now has a staple line and needs healing. Not eating the right foods can put pressure on the stomach that could cause a leakage. The post-op diet will provide the nutrients your body needs to heal quickly. This diet is in 5 phases or stages.

At each stage, you can assess how well you heal and from there proceed to the next diet stage. From the liquid stage, which is the first stage, the pureed, soft foods and to a final diet of protein-rich meals of low calories, you have all you need to maintain a healthy weight loss and achieve your health goals. Each stage is important and should not be skipped. You should spend at least a week in each stage. The post-op diet will make or mar your gastric sleeve surgery.

These 5 phases are:

1. **Phase 1 <u>Clear liquid</u>**

In this first phase, you will continue on the clear liquid diet that you were on days before the operation. This starts immediately after the surgery and last for about 7 days. Taking only clear liquids during this period is not hard; but rather a relief because most people do not even feel so hungry after their operation. The most important thing at this stage is not food, but staying hydrated.

2. **Phase 2A <u>Phase 2 Full Liquid</u>**

This diet is characterized by fuller liquids that are rich in protein. These are thin liquid foods that are not see-through. During this second week, you may have more appetite for food, but your digestive system isn't yet ready for solids. The full liquids may have a few chunks of solids in them. You should fill up on various nutritional liquids.

3. **Stage 2B- Pureed foods**

This phase is characterized by protein-packed purees. You should take about 60 grams of protein each day. Include protein in each meal by adding some milk when you blend. The mixture should be lump-free and must have a yoghurt-like consistency. It may be tough for you at this time, so it is best to eat small portions slowly so that body can have time to react. Watch out for foods that can upset your stomach and immediately avoid them. At this stage, it is also good to take supplements to prevent nutritional deficiencies.

4. **Stage 3- Soft foods**

From week 4-5, you can begin to introduce soft foods to your diet. These are tender foods that can be mashed and chewed easily. The purpose of this stage is to make it easy on the stomach to start digesting whole foods. You can also start to take caffeinated drinks in moderation. Aim to take 60 to 80 grams of protein per day and 56 to 64 ounces of fluid in a day. Each serving should consist of 1 to 2 ounces. Fish, eggs, beans and cooked vegetables should feature a lot during this phase and healthy fats from avocado.

5. **Stage 4- Solid foods**

At this stage, you can safely eat your solid foods. This new healthy eating plan should now become your new healthy eating pattern for life. A low fat, low calorie and portion controlled diet that will ensure your weight loss and health remains constant. Your diet should be rich in protein and vegetables of limited amounts. Eat 3 meals a day with minimal snacks and stay hydrated. New foods introduced should be monitored for any reaction. Steer clear of empty foods devoid of nutritional value. Avoid sugary sweets and sodas.

Major Rules Of Gastric Bypass Surgery Diet

There are rules that you must live by after your operation. These rules should be at your fingertips at all times. These are the things that you are allowed to do following a gastric bypass surgery. There are general guidelines for eating meals. Remember that you now have a small stomach with a capacity for a limited quantity of food.

1. Finish your meals before drinking anything. Drink only after 30 minutes after a meal.

2. Eat slowly. Each meal should take 20 to 30 minutes. During meals, eat your protein first, then your vegetables and then your carbs.

3. Chew food thoroughly. Larger pieces of food can block the narrow opening that leads from your stomach to your intestine. If foods stay too long in your stomach, you may experience nausea, vomiting and abdominal pain. If you can't chew, spit out. Don't swallow.

4. Keep to three small meals per day.

5. Avoid overeating. Once you feel full, stop eating. Overeating stretches your stomach pouch and can cause nausea and vomiting.

6. Introduce new foods one at a time, no more than one in a few days. New foods are foods you haven't eaten after your surgery even if you've had them before.

7. Don't snack between meals. Plan your meals and follow them. If you feel hungry between meals, try to take a drink. Your body may just need fluids and not food.

8. Drink lots of water.

9. Avoid unhealthy fats, processed or refined carbs and sugar.

10. Take recommended vitamin and mineral supplements.

Food Cravings After Gastric Surgery

Cravings pry on your mind and body in an attempt to make you eat something you shouldn't. Several things can cause cravings like boredom, stress, wrong environments and not planning meals well. After gastric bypass surgery, these cravings do not automatically go away. But they can be dealt with because it is all in the thoughts. After a while, your body will get used to it and you can fewer cravings by the day. So how do you prevent a craving from overpowering you?

1. Do not skip planned meals. If you do, you are giving room to cravings that may occur in the future. Be sure to eat regularly.

2. Discard unhealthy junk food from your pantry. You should do this before going for your surgery. Instead invest in healthy snacks such as smoothie, hard-boiled egg and fresh fruit yoghurt.

3. Stay hydrated. Drink water when you have cravings.

4. Reduce stress by sleeping well and exercising regularly. Stress causes our body to release the cortisol hormone which can increase hunger and cravings.

5. Resist sweets. Take dark chocolate when you crave a chocolate. But try to resist sweets generally because even those labeled sugar-free are high in fats and packed with calories.

6. Control your environment. Avoid places like the mall food courts and office vending machine. Limit your eating out and avoid fast foods restaurants.

7. Engage in healthy activities. Pick activities that you can do without eating. Walk your dog, wash your car. Look for something you like to do that will take your mind off food and cravings. Some of these may include: Running, taking a hike, going for a walk with a friend and walking your dog.

After gastric surgery, be prepared for a new way to eat. Your much smaller stomach will require new foods in smaller portions and within a particular time frame. Therefore, you will have to relearn and reintroduce foods at certain times. Even chewing foods will need to be relearnt! The best way to succeed in this diet is to listen to your body as what works for one may not work for the other. Be patient and be sure to consult with your dietician when in doubt.

Your stomach should heal naturally. With this diet also, you should also get used to eating smaller amounts of food. Your stomach can digest these smaller portions safety and comfortably. When you eat right, the diet will help you lose weight and avoid gaining them, avoid side effects and health issues, or complications from the operation.

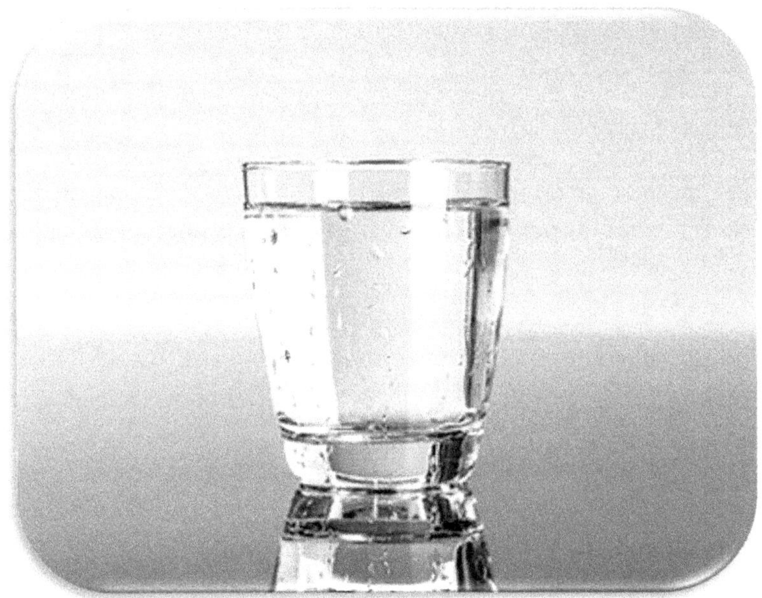

Pre-Op Meal Plan

Throughout your 2 to 3 weeks pre-operation meal plan, eat 5 times a day. Meals should include: 1 rich meal, 2 protein meal replacement shakes and sugar-free snacks. Total calories for women should not exceed 1200 while men may use up to about 1500 calories. For instance:

SAMPLE MEAL PLAN

Breakfast

One High Protein Shake (8-12 oz.) with a total calorie of less than 200

Snack

One non-starchy vegetable or fruit-based snack

Lunch/ Dinner

One main meal

Evening

One high protein shake

These meals are in no particular order and can be eaten in any order you wish. But ensure that you take at least 64 ounces of sugar-free fluids.

Liquids Allowed

- Water, flavored water
- Non-carbonated water like Fruit2O
- Fat-free broth (chicken, beef or vegetable)
- Sugar-free Popsicle's, Sugar-free Kool-Aid or Tang
- Smooth fruit

- Clear juices (without pulp or carbonation) e.g. apple, grape and cranberry
- Gelatin
- Sugar-free No cream coffee or tea (may include sugar substitutes)
- Almond milk

Suggestions For Protein Shakes

The pre-op diet is high in protein but low in carbohydrate; therefore you need high protein replacement meals. There are many protein shake brands on the market that are allowed on the pre-op diet but your total calories intake must than 200 less than 5 grams of sugar; but greater than 12 grams protein per serving.

These include:

- Slim Fast Low Carb
- Body Fortress Whey Protein Powder
- Atkins Shake
- Isopure
- Unjury
- ETB Naturally Protein
- Bariatric Advantage High Protein Meal
- GNC Pure Protein Shakes
- Boost Glucose control
- Designer Whey
- Celebrate ENS 4 in 1

They must be made from 100% whey protein isolate or whey protein.

Calories- >200

Protein- 15-25+ grams

Added sugar- 5-7 grams

Total fat- 4 grams and below

Snacks

Snacks daily Nutritional value is:

Calories - 100-250

Protein- 15-25+ grams

Added sugar- 5-7 grams

Total fat- 4 grams and below

Suggestions for snacks include:

- Low fat yogurt or light yogurt smoothie (less than 90 calories)
- Boiled egg
- Protein bars
- Detour Whey Protein Bar (170 calories)
- Pure Protein Bar (190-200 calories)
- Fiber One Protein Bar
- Protein shake
- ¼ cup of unsalted nuts
- ½ cup non-fat cottage cheese
- 1 cup non-starchy vegetables + 2 Tb hummus or guacamole
- 1 serving of fruit (150-250 calories)
- ½ pack of tuna
- 1 string cheese

Remember to wait for 30 minutes between foods and drinks.

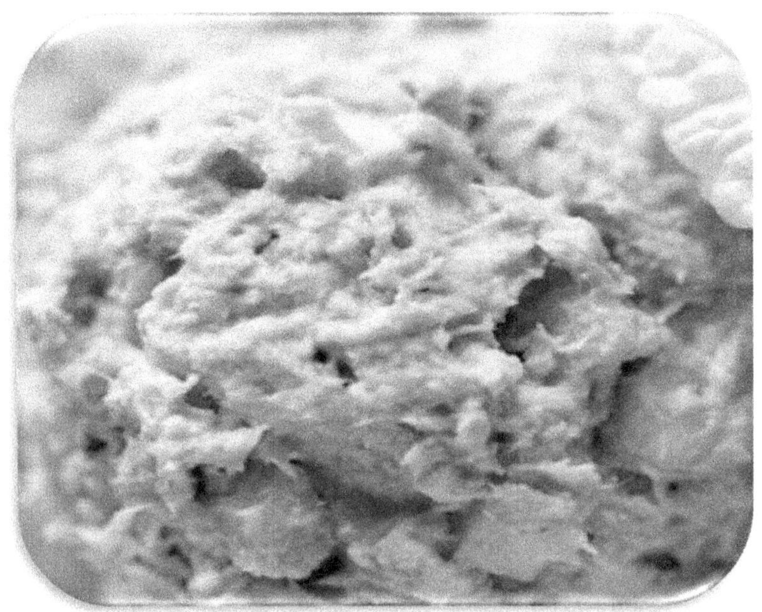

No Mayo Tuna Salad

Healthy, no mayo and flavorful, just the tuna salad you need!

Prep Time: 10 minutes

Total Time: 15 minutes

Servings: 6

Ingredients

4 5-oz. cans tuna, drained

2 stalks celery, thinly sliced

1/4 cup sliced green onion

1 carrot, shredded

1/2 red bell pepper, diced (about 1/4 cup)

1/4 cup extra-virgin olive oil

 2–3 tablespoons lemon juice

1 clove garlic, minced

1 tablespoon Dijon mustard

1/4 cup of fresh parsley, chopped

1/4 teaspoon kosher salt

Black pepper, to taste

Directions

1. Add the tuna to a large bowl and use a fork to flake.

2. Add the celery, green onion and carrot.

3. Combine the olive oil, juice of lemon, and garlic, mustard and fresh parsley in a bowl and once thoroughly mixed, add to the salad in the large bowl and stir to mix.

4. Add salt and pepper to taste and then serve.

Nutrition Per Serving: Calories 198; Fat 10.6g; Carbs 3.7g; Protein 22g; Fiber 1.1g; Sodium 471.4mg; Cholesterol 41.3mg

Oatmeal Raisin Cookie Shake

Prep Time: 3 minutes

Total Time: 3 minutes

Servings: 1

Ingredients

1 scoop whey powder, vanilla milkshake

1 tablespoon of quick oats

1 tablespoon of organic raisins

1/4 teaspoon of cinnamon

1 teaspoon of honey

1/3 cup of liquid egg whites (from 2 egg whites)

1 cup of vanilla almond milk, unsweetened

Directions

1. Place all the ingredients in a blender and blend thoroughly. Serve!

Nutrition Per Serving: Calories 311; Fat 6.4g; Carbs 21g; Protein 42g; Fiber 4.2g; Sodium 471.3mg; Cholesterol 95mg

Chicken & Apple Salad With Greens

Prep Time: 10 minutes

Total Time: 30 minutes

Servings: 3

Ingredients

For the Vinaigrette:

2 tablespoons of balsamic vinegar

2 tablespoons of orange juice

2 tablespoons of olive oil

1 tablespoon of lemon juice

1 tablespoon of reduced-sodium soy sauce

½ tablespoon Dijon mustard

½ tablespoon of brown sugar

¼ teaspoon of curry powder, optional

¼ teaspoon of salt

Pinch teaspoon pepper

Pinch teaspoon ground ginger

For The Salad:

1 cup of shredded cooked chicken

1 medium apples, chopped

14 cup red onion, thinly sliced

5 cups of torn mixed salad greens

¼ cup of toasted chopped walnuts

Directions

1. Place walnuts in a pan and bake in the oven for 5 to 10 minutes.

2. Place all the vinaigrette ingredients in a large bowl and whisk to blend.

3. Add the chicken and the apples and then the onions, toss all to coat.

4. To serve, place the salad greens on a serving platter. Add the chicken mixture on top and sprinkle with the walnuts.

Nutrition Per Serving: Calories 306; Fat 19g; Carbs 20g; Protein 17g; Fiber 4g; Sodium 549mg; Cholesterol 42mg

Zesty Shrimp Ceviche

Prep Time: I hour

Cook Time: 1 minute

Servings: 3

Ingredients

1 pound cooked shrimp cooked

¼ cup of red onion thinly sliced

1 small jalapeno

1/3 cup of cucumber diced

½ cup of Roma tomatoes

1/3 cup of cilantro leaves

1 small avocado

¼ cup of lime juice

2 tablespoons of lemon juice

1 tablespoon of orange juice

Salt to taste

Directions

1. Prepare your ingredients. Remove the ribs and seeds of the jalapeno and mince, dice the cucumber, chop the cilantro leaves and then seed and dice the tomatoes. Peel the avocado, seed and chop.

2. In a bowl, combine the shrimp, onion, jalapeno, tomatoes, and cucumber and cilantro.

3. Pour the lemon juice, lime juice and orange juice over it, season with salt and toss gently to incorporate.

4. Cover and chill 1 hour or overnight for 8 hours.

5. Just before serving, add the avocado

Nutrition Per Serving: Calories 236; Fat 3g; Carbs 1g; Protein 46g; Fiber 4g; Sodium 764mg; Cholesterol 571mg

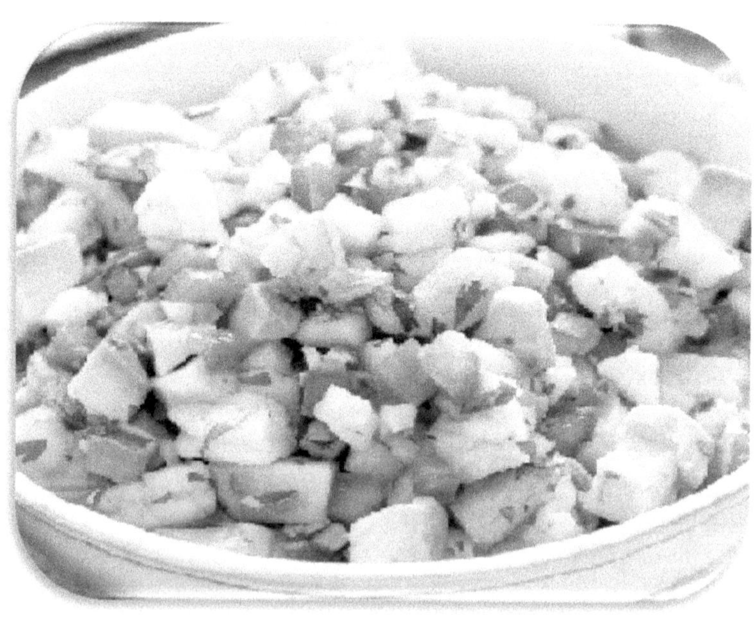

Quick Meatballs

Prep Time: 20 minutes

Cook Time: 15 minutes

Servings: 24 meatballs

Ingredients

2 large eggs

1/4 cup of water

1 small finely chopped onion

1-1/3 cups of soft bread crumbs

2/3 cup of Parmesan cheese, grated

2 garlic cloves, minced

2 teaspoons of Italian seasoning

1/4 teaspoon pepper

1 teaspoons salt

2 pounds ground beef

Directions

1. Preheat oven to 375°F.

2. Add together in a bowl, the eggs, water, bread crumbs, onion, the Parmesan cheese, the garlic and the seasonings. Mix thoroughly.

3. Add beef over mixture, crumble and thoroughly mix. Shape into balls of 1-1/2-inches. Place meatballs in shallow baking pans and transfer to greased racks.

4. Bake for 15 minutes, do not cover and remove once inside is no longer pinkish.

5. A serving is 3 meatballs. Freeze the rest in freezer containers. To use, place in the refrigerator overnight to thaw and heat in the microwave.

Nutrition Per Serving: Calories 276; Fat 17g; Carbs 6g; Protein 24g; Fiber 0g; Sodium 533mg; Cholesterol 122mg

Cream of Wheat Porridge

Prep Time: 5minutes

Cook Time: 3minutes

Servings: 2 (2 1/2 cups)

Ingredients

2 cups water

1 (3-inch) cinnamon stick

1/3 cup Cream of Wheat

Sugar and milk, to taste

Directions

1. Pour the water in a saucepan and add the cinnamon stick to it. Place the lid on the pot and bring the water to a boil.

2. Once the water boils, add the Cream of Wheat and stir with a whisk to make lump-free.

3. Lower heat and simmer, with the lid off, for 2 minutes or until thickened.

4. Remove saucepan from heat, discard the cinnamon stick.

5. Add milk and sugar to sweeten and stir to incorporate well.

Nutrition Per Serving: Calories 295; Fat 22g; Carbs 16g; Protein 9g; Fiber 2g; Sodium 116mg; Cholesterol 69mg

Citrus Salmon With Quinoa Salad

Looks good, smells great and tastes delicious, it will make you feel great as well!

Prep Time: 20 minutes

Cook Time: 15 minutes

Servings: 4

Ingredients

¾ cup of uncooked quinoa

½ cup of carrots, grated

¼ cup chopped parsley

½ cup of chopped capsicum

¼ cup of chopped coriander

1 Spanish onion

1 teaspoon of lime juice

1 teaspoon of lemon juice

1 tablespoon of orange juice

2 garlic cloves

2 tablespoon of olive oil

1 tablespoon of tamari soy sauce

1 teaspoon fresh ginger

1 teaspoon of fresh chili

1 tablespoon of low fat yoghurt

<u>Marinade</u>

1 tablespoon of lemon juice

1 tablespoon of lime juice

1 teaspoon lemon zest

1 teaspoon lime zest

1 teaspoon orange zest

1 tablespoon of orange juice

4(6-7 ounce) salmon

Directions

1. Rinse the quinoa and drain, place in a saucepan. Add 2 cups of water to the pan and bring to a boil. Cover and let it simmer for 15 minutes, or until the water is absorbed. Remove and set aside for 10 minutes. Fluff with a fork.

2. In a large bowl, add together the carrot, parsley, capsicum, the coriander and the Spanish onion. Add the cooled quinoa and mix.

3. Whisk together the orange, lime and lemon juices, the ginger, tamari, garlic and the chilli. Pour over the salad and mix thoroughly.

4. Combine the citrus marinade dressing and the salmon in a bowl. Set aside for 15 minutes to marinate.

5. Pan-fry the salmon lightly until slightly pink in the middle.

6. Serve salmon on the Quinoa salad and top with a little low fat yoghurt.

Nutrition Per Serving: Calories 166.3; Fat 37g; Carbs 50g; Protein 46g; Fiber 0g; Sodium 397mg;

Sticky Garlic Sesame Chicken

Prep Time: 5 minutes

Cook Time: 20 minutes

Servings: 3

Ingredients

1/4 cup of flour

1/2 teaspoon onion

1/8 teaspoon red pepper

1/4 teaspoon pepper

1 pound chicken tenders, cut into pieces

2 tablespoons extra virgin oil, olive

1/4 cup + 1 tablespoon honey

1 teaspoon rice vinegar

3 tablespoons of soy sauce

2 large cloves garlic, minced

1/8 teaspoon red pepper flakes

4 green onions (chopped)

1/2 teaspoon of sesame seeds

1 1/2 cups of rice

Directions

1. Add oil to pan and heat.

2. In a large Ziploc bag, add together the flour, the red pepper, and the onion powder. Shake and add the chicken pieces to it. Shake bag again to coat thoroughly.

3. Remove coated chicken pieces carefully to pan and cook on both sides for 10 minutes until browned.

4. In the meantime, add together in a small dish: the honey, minced garlic, rice vinegar, together with the red pepper flakes, and soy sauce. Whisk to mix and set to one side.

5. Add the sauce mix to the browned chicken in the pan, set heat to low and heat for 10 minutes, but turn over once.

6. Prepare the rice.

7. Turn off stove and let it rest for 5 minutes. Add a sprinkling of sesame seeds to top and add some chopped green onions as well.

Nutrition Per Serving: Calories 128; Fat 17g; Carbs 9g; Protein 1g; Sodium 4mg;

Lean Burgers

Amazingly juicy!

Prep Time: 20minutes

Cook Time: 20minutes

Servings: 4

Ingredients

1 slice whole-grain bread, torn into 1-inch squares

2 tablespoons of milk

1 lb. extra-lean ground beef

Salt, freshly ground black pepper, to taste

4 1-oz slices Swiss cheese

4 whole-wheat hamburger buns

1 teaspoon olive oil

1/2 sweet onion, sliced

Directions

1. Preheat oven to 350°F.

2. Line a rimmed baking sheet with aluminum foil. Spritz with cooking spray.

3. Add bread to a small bowl. Add milk gradually; 1/2 tablespoon at a time. Make a paste.

4. Place beef in a separate but bigger bowl. Add the bread-milk paste and use your hands to work into beef thoroughly. Season with salt and pepper or any other desired burger seasonings. Form mixture into 4 patties.

5. Place burgers on baking sheet on a bottom rack and cook for 15 minutes, flipping once. About 2 minutes to end of cooking time, top with 1 slice cheese each

6. Place the buns on top rack to enable them toast. Do not let them burn.

7. Meanwhile, sauté onion in until tender. Remove and set aside.

8. Remove cooked burgers from the bottom of the rack in the oven, place on toasted buns and top with cooked onion.

Nutrition Per Serving: Calories 328; Fat 10g; Carbs 26g; Protein 35g; Fiber 4g; Sodium 405mg; Cholesterol 70mg

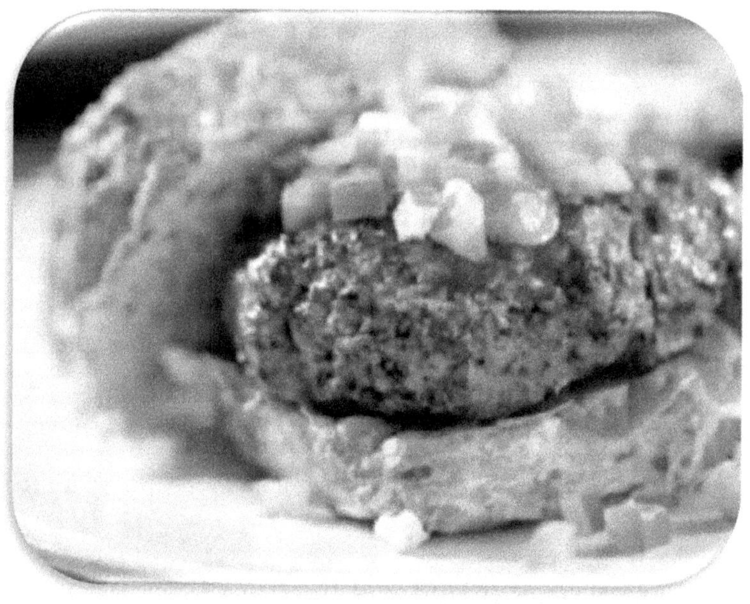

Egg And Potato Breakfast Scramble

An easy, versatile, breakfast filled of scrambled eggs, herbs and cheese!

Prep Time: 10minutes

Cook Time: 15minutes

Servings: 2

Ingredients

6 ounces red potatoes (from 4 small red potatoes), rinsed, scrubbed and diced.

¼ cup water

2 teaspoons extra virgin olive oil

Pinch salt

3 large eggs, beaten

Dash of milk

1 scallion, thinly sliced

⅓cup of grated Gruyère cheese

1 tablespoon freshly chopped thyme

Directions

1. Add together the potatoes, the water, oil and salt in a non- stick pan. Cover, set heat to high and bring to a boil. Cook 5 minutes.

2. Once the water evaporates and the potatoes begin to sauté, uncover and loosen from the bottom with a wooden spoon. Brown for 5 minutes

3. Scramble the eggs with milk in a bowl. Pour into the pan, add the scallions and scramble well until the eggs are just set. Remove from heat.

4. Sprinkle with grated cheese and thyme. Let it sit to melt for a minute. Enjoy!

Nutrition Per Serving: Calories 465; Fat 18.1g; Carbs 55.7g; Protein 21.6g; Fiber 6.1g; Sodium 446mg; Cholesterol 298mg

STAGE 1- Clear Liquids Meal Plan

Clear liquid diet is usually a continuation of the liquid diet you had 2 to3 days before surgery. However, the most important thing at this stage is to stay hydrated. Spread fluids consumption throughout the day. Drink from the time you get up in the morning and throughout the day until you go to bed. Every hour, take 1-2 ounces of clear liquid. Sipping water will prevent nausea as well. Sip liquids continuously (64 ounces (6-8) cups of fluids).

Suggestions For Clear Liquid:

- Light or diluted fruit juices such as apple, grape, cranberry fruit juice; no more than 2 cups per day.
- water, ice chips popsicles, non-carbonated flavored waters
- broths
- gelatin (all sugar free)
- diluted sugar-free squash
- 1percent milk

SAMPLE MEAL PLAN

<u>**Breakfast**</u>

Water

<u>**Snacks**</u>

Fat-free milk, flavored water

Lunch

Apple juice; sugar-free jello

Dinner

Fat-free bro

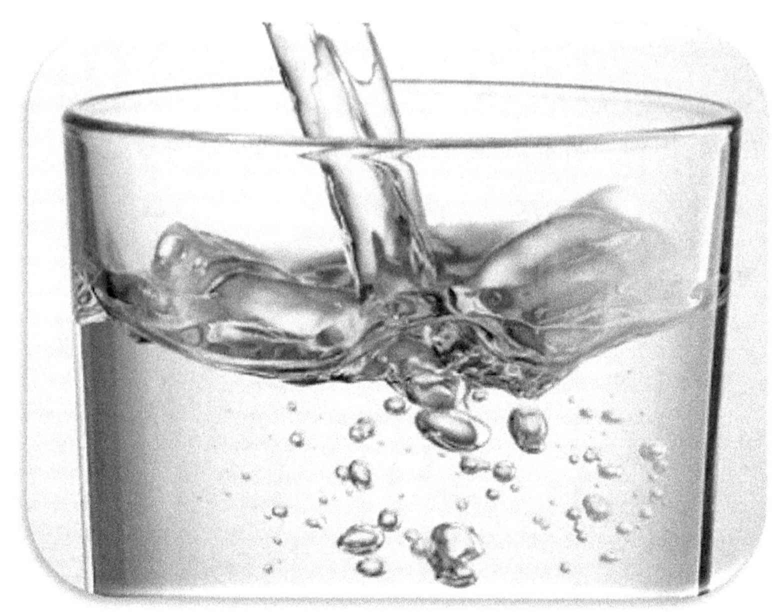

Some Tea Recipes

Peanut & Ginger Tea

Prep Time: 2 minutes

Total Time: 10 minutes

Servings: 2

Ingredients

2 cups of water

20 dry unsalted roasted peanuts

4 slices fresh ginger root (1/4 inch thickness)

Directions

1. Shell the peanuts and chop coarsely.

2. Bring water to a boil.

3. Add the chopped peanuts and the ginger to the water and immediately remove from heat.

4. Let it steep for 5 minutes. Pass tea through a strainer and transfer to two cups.

5. Add a teaspoon of artificial sweetener, if recommended, into each cup, stir and serve.

Nutrition Per Serving: Calories 81; Fat 5g; Carbs 8g; Protein 3g; Cholesterol 0mg; Sodium 12mg

Wild Peppermint Tea

Prep Time: 2 minutes

Total Time: 37 minutes

Servings: 4

Ingredients

½cup of peppermint leaf, dry or fresh

3 cups boiling water

Directions

1. Bring the water to boil and then add the peppermint leaves and let it steep for 5 minutes or thereabouts.

2. Strain tea, add sweetener, if recommended and pour tea into cups.

Nutrition Per Serving: Calories 34.2; Fat 0g; Carbs 9g; Protein 1g; Cholesterol 0mg; Sodium 5mg

Lavender Mint Tea

Preparation Time: 0 minutes

Total Time: 5 minutes

Servings: 1

Ingredients

2 teaspoons fresh lavender flowers or 1 teaspoon dried lavender flowers

1 1/2-2 tablespoons of fresh mint leaves or 2 teaspoons dried mint

1 cup boiling water

Directions

1. Place the herbs in a tea ball or brew in tea and then strain.

2. Pour boiling water over the herbs and let it steep for 5 minutes. If needed, strain and serve it hot. Sweeten, if desired.

3. To make as iced tea, double the amount of herbs and let it steep overnight in a quart of water. Refrigerate and add more water, if desired. Also, sweeten, if desired.

Nutrition Per Serving: Calories 2.8; Fat 0g; Carbs 0.5g; Protein 0.2g; Cholesterol 0mg; Sodium 8mg

Some Infused Water Recipes

Blueberry/ Mint Infused Waters

Ingredients

2 cups of blueberries

2 sprigs mint, muddled

2 quarts water

Directions

1. Place the muddled mint, blueberries and water in a container.

2. Stir and refrigerate 4 hours or overnight.

Cherry Minty

Ingredients

1 sprig of mint

1 Key lime, thinly sliced

6 pitted cherries cut in1/2

Directions

1. Combine and let it steep for 30 minutes.

2. Chill or serve it over ice.

Ingredients

8 large strawberries, thinly sliced

1 cucumber, thinly sliced

2 limes, juiced

Directions

1. Add together all the ingredients in a pitcher.

2. Add cold water, cover, and store in the refrigerator overnight.

Citrus Mix

Ingredients

1 lime, sliced thinly

1 orange, sliced thinly

1/2 of a lemon, thinly sliced

2 quarts of water

Directions

1. Add the lime, orange and lemon to the water Refrigerate for at least4 hours.

2. Serve over ice, garnished with 1 sprig of basil.

Some Simple Broth/ Soups

Simple Chicken Broth

Prep Time: 10 minutes

Cook Time: 45 minutes

Servings: 8 cups

Ingredients

1 chicken breast

1/2 teaspoon salt

1 teaspoon extra virgin olive oil

1 large red onion, peeled, chopped

2 stalks celery, trimmed chopped

2 medium carrots, peeled, chopped

1/4 cup parsley, chopped

1 teaspoon of whole black peppercorns

2 bay leaves

12 cups of water

Directions

1. Sprinkle the chicken with sea salt.

2. Cook the chicken in a large stockpot for 4 minutes. Cook with the skin side down until browned.

3. Add the carrots, onions, and celery in the pot and cook another 4 minutes, with occasional stirring.

4. Add the peppercorns, parsley and the bay leaf. Pour the water and bring to a boil gently. Let the heat be high. Reduce heat and simmer for 25 minutes. Use a spoon to skim fat off the top of the broth.

5. Remove the chicken, discard the skin and set aside meat for future use.

6. Let the broth cool completely and then store refrigerated in an air-tight bowl. Store for up to a week or in the freezer for up to 6 months.

7. Before using, discard the bay leaf and peppercorns. Serving Size: 1 cup

Nutrition Per Serving: Calories 40; Fat 2g; Carbs 4g; Protein 0g; Fiber 1g; Sodium 125mg; Cholesterol 1mg

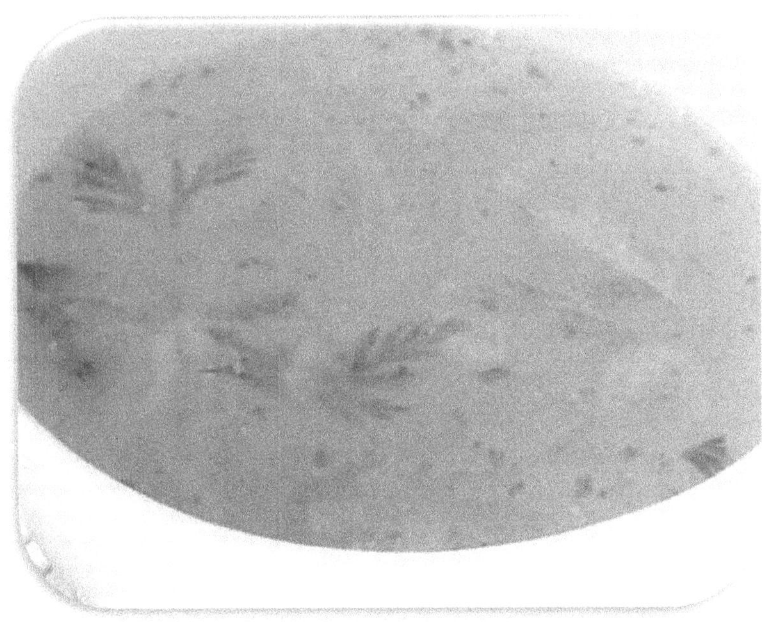

No Potato Clam Chowder

Prep Time: 10minutes

Total Time: 35 minutes

Servings: 4

Ingredients

3.5 ounce clams

2 tablespoons of butter

5 ounce un-smoked bacon or pancetta, cubed

1 onion, finely chopped

1 bay leaf

Sprig of thyme

1 tablespoon of plain flour

¾ cup of milk

¾ cup of double cream

Directions

1. Rinse the clams several times and drain. Add to a large pan of 2 cups of water and bring to a boil.

2. Simmer for 2 minutes. Once the clams have opened, pour onto a colander over a bowl of water and let it cool. Now take out the clams from their shells and strain unto a bowl until you have about 3 to 31/2 stock.

3. Heat the butter in same pan, add the bacon and cook for a few minutes until brown. Add the onion, thyme and the bay leaf and cook for 10 minutes until the onions is translucent.

4. Spread the flour over it and stir for 2 minutes until sandy. Add the clam stock gradually, and then add the milk and the cream.

Nutrition Per Serving: Calories 433; Fat 29g; Carbs 19g; Protein 22g; Fiber 2g;

STAGE 2A- Full Liquids Meal Plan

At this stage, your diet is protein-packed. Eat smaller meals throughout the day, about 5-6 meals daily. These meals should consist of 1-2 tablespoons per meal and you can increase it gradually to 4 four tablespoons. Include protein in each meal. Blended foods should also include a pint of milk. Remember to sip slowly and do not use straws.

Protein = 60-70 grams

Water= 64 ounces

Full Liquid Choices Include:

- Thin broth/smooth soups (no chunks) such as cream of tomato, or oxtail
- Blended fruit juices (no pulp)
- Skimmed milk, Unsweetened Milk
- Homemade smoothies
- Yogurt drinks (nonfat plain Greek yogurt)
- Protein powder shakes
- No-sugar nutrition shakes (Ensure Light)
- Sugar-free, nonfat pudding
- Sorbet
- Thinned, hot cereal, such as oatmeal
- Soft egg-based products

<u>Avoid At This Stage</u>

- Solid foods
- High-fat foods
- Sugary foods
- Foods with seeds
- Food with lump

- Cheese, tofu, noodles, rice
- Whole fruits and vegetables

SAMPLE MEAL PLAN

<u>Breakfast</u>

Cooked cereal (oatmeal)

<u>Snack</u>

Yogurt smoothie

<u>Lunch/ Dinner</u>

Pureed soup

<u>Desserts and Snacks</u>

Milkshakes, sherbet, custard-style yogurt, pudding, gelatin with whipped cream fruit juice bars etc.

Note that you can rotate different types of cereals and juices. You can make your liquids more protein-packed by adding protein powder or skim milk powder to it. Meal replacement drinks also help. When you take soups, you can take some a cup or glass of tea, milk or vegetable juice to go along with it.

Blueberry Avocado Protein Smoothie

Get fuller and longer with this smoothie that's packed with protein and healthy fats.

Prep Time: 5 minutes

Total Time: 10 minutes

Servings: 1

Ingredients

1/2 medium avocado

1 cup frozen blueberries

1 cup of unsweetened almond milk

1/3 cup of egg whites

1 small scoop of stevia extract

1 scoop of vanilla protein powder

Directions

1. Blend all the ingredients in a Vitamix blender. Serve!

Nutrition Per Serving: Calories 388; Fat 14.3g; Carbs 29.3g; Protein 35.4g; Fiber 13.2g; Sodium 350.5mg; Cholesterol 5mg

Simple Chocolate Protein Pudding

The perfect afternoon snack or dessert!

Prep Time: 5 minutes

Total Time: 5 minutes

Servings: 1

Ingredients

1 serving vegan chocolate protein powder

2 tablespoons of or cocoa powder

1 cup of chilled non- dairy milk

1 tablespoon almond butter

Directions

1. Add together the protein powder, the cocoa powder and ¾ cup of preferred dairy-free milk in a bowl; stir to remove most of the lumps. Add the remaining milk.

2. Now add the creamy almond butter to the lump-free pudding and stir thoroughly.

3. Place on the refrigerator to thicken or serve immediately. Shelf life in the refrigerator is up to 8 hours.

Nutrition Per Serving: Calories 239; Fat 13g; Carbs 17g; Protein 21g; Fiber 10g;

Banana Protein Pudding

Prep Time: 5 minutes

Total Time: 5 minutes

Servings: 2

Ingredients

1 ripe banana, mashed

1 scoop of Vanilla Whey Protein

11/4 cup of Greek yogurt

1/2 teaspoon of cinnamon

2 teaspoons of honey

1/2 teaspoon of vanilla extract

<u>Toppings</u>

Sliced banana, almond butter

Directions

1. Combine all the ingredients and blend until smooth.

2. Place in a jar and top as desired.

3. Refrigerate and serve as breakfast or dessert.

Nutrition Per Serving: w/o toppings Calories 289; Fat 10g; Carbs 44g; Protein 24g;

Slow Cooker Oatmeal

Prep Time: 2 minutes

Total Time: 2 minutes

Servings: 2

Ingredients

3 cups water

1 cup old-fashioned rolled oats

1/4 cup of half-and-half

Splenda brown sugar to taste

Directions

1. Add the oats and water in a slow cooker and stir to mix.

2. Place lid on and cook 8 hours on low or overnight.

3. Add the half-and-half and season with brown sugar. Stir gently and serve with more cream.

Nutrition Per Serving: Calories 178; Fat 6.9g; Carbs 27.5g; Protein 3.1g; Fiber 1.9g; Sodium 17.2mg;

High Protein Vanilla Pudding

Prep Time: 2 minutes

Total Time: 2 minutes

Servings: 1

Ingredients

3/4 cup of plain Greek yogurt

1 scoop vanilla brown rice protein powder

1-11/2 tablespoons of coconut flour

Directions

1. Add yogurt to a bowl. Add the protein powder and mix to fully incorporate.

2. Add the flour, mix well to desired consistency.

3. Refrigerate to thicken or enjoy immediately.

Nutrition Per Serving: w/o toppings Calories 180; Fat 1g; Carbs 14g; Protein 31g;

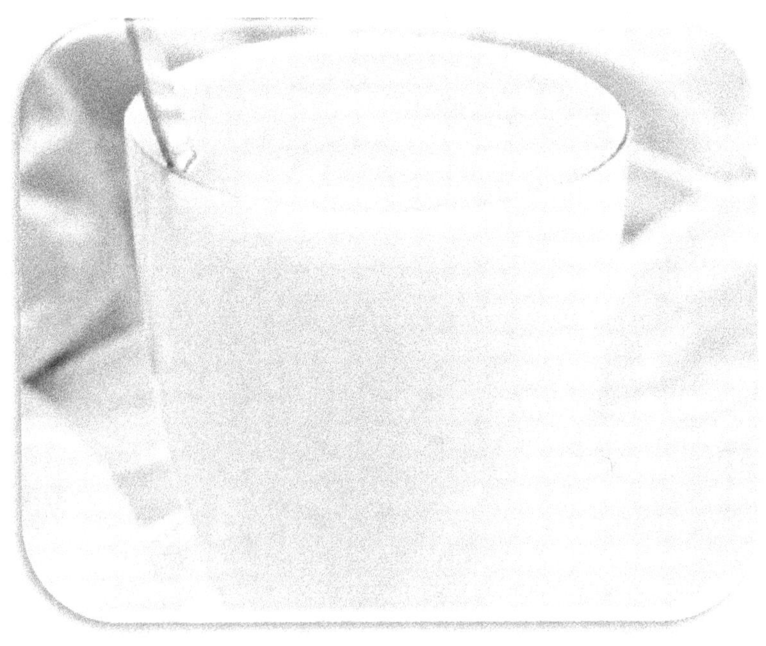

Light Berry Frozen Yogurt

Prep Time: 15 minutes

Total Time: 15minutes

Servings: 6

Ingredients

2 cups frozen berries

1 cup of plain yogurt

1/2 cup of 1%milk

1 cup ice

4 droppers of vanilla liquid stevia

Directions

1. Blend all ingredients together.

2. Add mixture to an ice cream machine and prepare as directed in the manual.

3. Alternatively, pour into a container, cover tightly and freeze for 3 hours. This mixture makes 24 ounces of yoghurt.

Nutrition Per Serving: Calories 76; Fat 3g; Carbs 10g; Protein 3g; Fiber 1g;

Peanut Applesauce Chicken

Prep Time: 10 minutes

Cook Time: 1 hour

Servings: 8

Ingredients

2½ lb. chicken pieces

¼ cup of yellow mustard

½ cup of powdered peanuts

⅛ cup Splenda brown sugar

Salt and pepper to taste

1 (15 oz.) jar applesauce, unsweetened

Directions

1. Place the chicken in a pan and sauté until brown.

2. At the last 5 minutes of cooking, add the rest of the ingredients and stir well to incorporate.

3. Simmer and remove once internal temperature registers 165°F

Nutrition Per Serving(2 tablespoons): Calories 50; Fat 2g; Carbs 13g; Protein 3g; Fiber 2g; Sodium 203mg; Cholesterol: 60 mg

Egg Drop Soup

Prep Time: 2 minutes

Total Time: 5 minutes

Servings: 1

Ingredients

1 egg

1/8 teaspoon of freshly ground black pepper

11/2 cup of clear chicken broth

1 teaspoon low-sodium soy sauce

1 large green onion, chopped (only the green parts)

Directions

1. Whisk the egg in a small bowl, along with the black pepper.

2. Add the broth and soy sauce to a pan and heat over medium high heat. Add the egg slowly into the boiling broth and let it set. Now whisk with a fork, gently.

3. Remove, transfer to a soup bowl, add the chopped green onions to garnish and serve.

Nutrition Per Serving: Calories 93; Fat 5g; Carbs 3.6g; Protein 8g; Fiber 0.7g; Sodium 836mg;

STAGE 2B- Pureed Foods Meal Plan

Daily protein intake - 60 grams. Eat 3 small meals each day. Take protein supplements after each meal.

Food suggestion for protein- packed foods

- Yogurt
- Strained cream soups
- Mashed cottage cheese
- Ricotta cheese
- Scrambled eggs
- Pureed beef or chicken
- Thick blended soups
- White fish, mashed or blended steamed fish
- Mashed sweet potato
- Tomato juice
- Pureed peaches, pears, apricots
- Applesauce

SAMPLE MEAL PLAN

Eat protein first, and liquids 30 minutes between meals.

Breakfast

1/4 cup scrambled egg

2 tablespoon of wheat

Lunch

2 tablespoon cottage cheese (low fat)

Mashed sweet potato

<u>**Snack/ Dessert**</u>

2 tablespoon of purred peaches with juice

<u>**Dinner**</u>

1/4 cup pureed chicken breast

1/4 cup mashed avocado

Avoid At This Stage:

- Pureed fibrous vegetables such as broccoli, celery, asparagus and cauliflower
- High starchy foods like bread and pasta
- Spicy foods
- Fatty foods

PUREED FOOD RECIPES

Healthy Soft Scrambled Eggs

Prep Time: 2 minutes

Cook Time: 3 minutes

Servings: 2

Ingredients

4 eggs

1/2 tablespoon of butter

Salt to taste

Directions

1. Add the butter to a non-stick skillet and melt over medium low heat.

2. Add whisked egg to the bubbling butter. Add to the centre. Once the edges starts to set, stir the edges gently to make soft curds but do not flip over curds. Keep at it for 2 minutes until the eggs are barely set.

4. Remove soft scrambled eggs from heat. Enjoy!

Nutrition Per Serving: Calories 168; Fat 12.4g; Carbs 0.7g; Protein 12.6g; Cholesterol 379.6mg; Sodium 142.4mg

Homemade Tomato Juice

Prep Time: 5 minutes

Total Time: 5 minutes

Servings: 2

Ingredients

4 medium tomatoes

1 cucumber

1 stalk celery

1/4 red bell pepper

Freshly ground black pepper

1/2 teaspoon sea salt

Cayenne pepper

Lemon wedges

Directions

1. Wash vegetables. Remove the stem and seeds from the bell pepper and chop largely.

2. Process vegetables and herbs in a food processor.

3. Season with salt and pepper, as well as the cayenne pepper as desired. Stir to mix all.

4. Refrigerate and serve. Garnish juice with lemon wedges.

Nutrition Per Serving: Calories 87; Fat 1g; Carbs 20g; Protein 4g; Fiber 5g; Sodium 519mg; Cholesterol 1mg

Crockpot Cinnamon Roll Oatmeal

Prep Time: 5 minutes

Cook Time: 2 hours

Servings: 4

Ingredients

2 cups gluten-free oats

2 eggs

3 cups almond milk

1/2 cup of sugar

2 tablespoons of flour or baking mix, gluten-free

1 teaspoon of vanilla

1 teaspoon of cinnamon

Glaze

1 cup of powdered sugar

2 tablespoons of milk

1/4 teaspoon of vanilla extract

Directions

1. Add together all the ingredients in a crockpot. Set to cook for 4 hours on low temperature or 2 hours on high.

2. Once done, open and transfer oatmeal to bowls.

3. Add together the glaze ingredients and drizzle to served oatmeal bowls.

Nutrition Per Serving: Calories 549; Fat 12g; Carbs 97g; Protein 15g; Fiber 5g; Sodium 209mg;Cholesterol 101mg

Millet & Pumpkin Congee

A hearty, whole grain breakfast!

Prep Time: 5 minutes

Cook Time: 30 minutes

Servings: 4

Ingredients

1/2 cup of millet

2 cups of pumpkin cubes

8 cups water

Brown sugar to taste

Directions

1. Peel the pumpkin, cut it into small cubes and place in a pot. Let it cook until softened. This should take about 10 minutes. Once cooked, smash it.

2. Wash the millet and add to the smashed pumpkin in the pot. Cover and let it boil over high heat. Reduce heat to medium and then cook for an additional 15 minutes, stirring occasionally.

3. Add the sugar. Serve!

Nutrition Per Serving: Calories 109; Fat 1g; Carbs 21g; Protein 3g; Fiber 2g; Sodium 26mg

Italian Chicken Soup

Prep Time: 10 minutes

Cook Time: 45 minutes

Servings: 2

Ingredients

1/2 fennel bulb, chopped

1/4 cup of chopped onion

1 teaspoons canola oil

1 cup hot water

2 cups low sodium chicken broth

3/4 cups of carrots, chopped

1/8 teaspoon dried basil

1/8 teaspoon dried thyme

1/8 teaspoon pepper

1/8 teaspoon salt

1 cup cooked chicken breast, cubed

1/4 cup of uncooked orzo pasta

1 tablespoon fennel fronds, finely chopped

Directions

1. Add the fennel bulb and chopped onion in oil and sauté until softened.

2. Add the chicken broth, carrots, basil, thyme, pepper, salt and the cooked chicken breast. Bring to a boil. Se heat to low and simmer for about 15 minutes.

3. Add the chicken and orzo and stir to mix. Cover and let it cook for 20 minutes.

4. Once the orzo is soft, add the fennel fronds.

Nutrition Per Serving: Calories 279; Fat 5g; Carbs 30g; Protein 28g; Fiber 1.1g; Sodium 829mg; Cholesterol 54mg

Chocolate Porridge

Prep Time: 10 minutes

Cook Time: 10 minutes

Servings: 1

Ingredients

1/3 cup rolled oats

1/3 cup almond milk

1/3 cup water

1 ripe banana, mashed

2 teaspoon cocoa powder

1/2 tablespoon of preferred sweetener

1 teaspoon of coconut oil

Optional Toppings - fruit, berries, cacao nibs, chocolate chips, nut butter, etc.

Directions

1. Combine oats, milk and water in a pan. Set heat on medium high and cook mixture until bubbling.

2. Lower heat and then add the mashed banana, cocoa powder, sweetener and oil. Let it simmer for 5 to 10 minutes or to desired consistency.

3. Top porridge with berries and nut, drizzled with tahini. Serve!

Nutrition Per Serving: w/o toppings: Calories 304; Fat 8g; Carbs 56g; Protein 7.2g; Fiber 8.2g;

Roasted Acorn Squash Soup

A smooth and delightful soup of roasted acorn squash blended with other healthy ingredients.

Prep Time: 20 minutes

Cook Time: 1hr 5 minutes

Servings: 3

Ingredients

1 acorn squash, halved &seeded

¼ cup of water, as needed

11/2 tablespoons of unsalted butter

1 small sweet onion, chopped

1 small carrot, peeled, then chopped

1 small clove garlic, minced

1½ - 2 cups of low-sodium chicken stock

1/8 cup half-and-half

1/4 teaspoon ground cinnamon

1/4 teaspoon ground nutmeg

Salt and ground black pepper to taste

Directions

1. Preheat oven to 400 F

2. Place the squash in a baking pan, ensuring that the cut side faces down. Add water to the baking dish, let enough water to cover the bottom

3. Bake in the oven for 45 minutes or thereabouts and remove once a fork can pierce the flesh of the squash. Scoop the flesh in a bowl.

4. Now melt the butter in a pot and add the onion, carrot and the minced garlic in the melted butter. Cook for 5 minutes or a little more and then pour the chicken stock in the pot. This is the time to add the squash and cook for 20- 25 minutes.

5. Transfer mixture to a blender and pulse. Puree in batches, if necessary, until smooth. Return blended soup to pot.

6. Add the half-and-half, cinnamon and nutmeg in the pot. Season with salt and pepper. Add a little more water to thin the soup.

Nutrition Per Serving: Calories 155.4; Fat 7.5g; Carbs 21g; Protein 3.9g; Fiber 5.8g; Sodium 125.3mg; Cholesterol 21.3mg

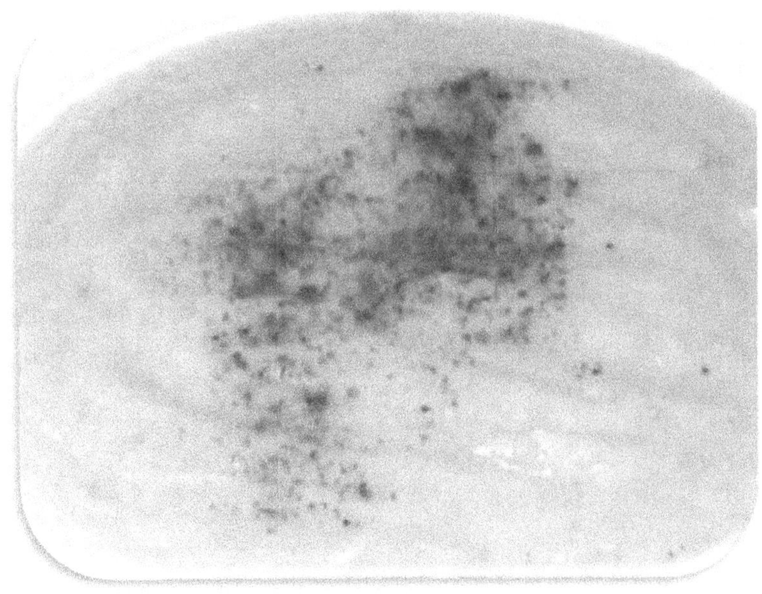

Garlic Mashed Cauliflower

Prep Time: 15 minutes

Cook Time: 10 minutes

Servings: 4

Ingredients

1 head cauliflower, cut into florets

1 tablespoon canola oil

1 clove garlic, smashed

¼ cup mozzarella cheese, grated

1 tablespoon of low-fat cream cheese

½ teaspoon salt

1/8 teaspoon fresh ground black pepper

Directions

1. Place a steamer insert into a saucepan. Add water to it to fill below the bottom of the steamer. Let it boil. Add the cauliflower to the pan and cover. Steam for 10 minutes until tender.

2. Add olive oil to a skillet and heat. Add the garlic and cook 2 minutes to soften. Remove

3. Blend ½ of the cauliflower in a food processor. Add the remaining florets gradually, garlic, cheese, cream cheese and the salt and pepper. Blend until creamy.

Nutrition Per Serving: Calories 98; Fat 5.7g; Carbs 8.4g; Protein 5.2g; Fiber 3.6g; Sodium 372mg; Cholesterol 7mg

Curried Coconut Chicken Soup

A spicy, sweet and filling recipe.

Prep Time: 15 minutes

Cooking time: 35 minutes

Servings: 4

Ingredients:

1 can of light coconut milk

2 chicken breasts, skinless, boneless

5 cups of chicken stock

2 cups of cauliflower florets, chopped

½ cup of fresh cilantro, chopped

1 garlic clove, crushed

1 small onion, chopped

1 lime, juiced

2 tablespoons of coconut oil

2 tablespoons of curry powder

Salt

Pepper

Shredded coconut

Directions:

1. Heat a large pot over medium heat and add the oil.

2. Sauté the onion until softened.

3. Add the garlic and sauté for another minute.

4. Stir in the curry powder and cauliflower; cook for an additional minute.

5. Add pepper and salt to season.

6. Add the chicken and stock; give it time to boil and lower heat to a simmer for 20 minutes until the chicken is well cooked and the cauliflower soft.

7. Transfer chicken to a cutting board and shred with two forks.

8. Return shredded chicken to pot and stir in the lime juice, cilantro and coconut milk. Simmer for 5-10 minutes until well heated.

9. Top with shredded coconut and serve hot.

Nutrition Per Serving: Calories 374; Fat 27g; Carbs 10g; Protein 24g; Fiber 4g;

Italian Chicken Puree

Prep Time: 10 minutes

Cook Time: 0 minute

Servings: 1

Ingredients

1/4 cup of canned chicken

1 1/2 tablespoon of tomato sauce

1/8 teaspoon of pepper

1/8 teaspoon of salt

1teaspoon of Italian seasoning

Directions

1. Blend all the ingredients in a blender. Blend well until soft.

2. Transfer to a bowl and microwave for 35 seconds.

Nutrition Per Serving: Fat 4g; Carbs 3g; Protein 13g;

Easy 3-Ingredient Tomato Soup

Velvety, rich 3- ingredient tomato soup recipe.

Prep Time: 5 minutes

Total Time: 40 minutes

Servings: 2

Ingredients

4 tablespoons of unsalted butter

1/2 onion, cut largely into wedges

1 (28-oz) can tomatoes

1 1/2 cups water or stock

1/2 teaspoon salt

Directions

1. Melt the butter in a saucepan

2. Add the wedges of onion, water or low sodium stock, can of tomatoes, inclusive of juices, and the salt.

3. Let it simmer and then cover. Cook for 40 minutes with occasional stirring.

4. Blend soup with an immersion blender.

Nutrition Per Serving: Calories 348; Fat 24.9g; Carbs 29.6g; Protein7.8;Fiber 4.5g; Cholesterol 61mg; Sodium 1485.4mg

White Bean Puree

Prep Time: 7 minutes

Cook Time: 15minutes

Servings: 4

Ingredients

3 tablespoons of unsalted butter

1 small onion, diced well

1 clove garlic, minced

1 thyme sprig

2(15-oz.) cans cannellini beans, drained &rinsed

1 cup chicken broth, low-sodium

Salt and ground pepper

Directions

1. Melt the butter in a saucepan and then add the onion, the minced garlic and then the thyme spring. Let it cook for about 7 minutes. Stir constantly and remove once the onion is tender.

2. Add the beans, pour in the broth and cook 5 minutes or until the broth is lessened by half. Throw away the sprig.

3. Puree in an immersion blender and add salt and pepper to taste. Enjoy while still hot.

Pureed Chicken Salad

Prep Time: 10 minutes

Cook Time: 5minutes

Servings: 1

Ingredients

1 chicken breast cooked

2 tablespoons of Greek yogurt

2 tablespoons light mayonnaise

1/8 teaspoon onion powder

1/8 teaspoon celery salt

Pinch black pepper

Directions

1. Process the chicken breast in a food processor.

2. Pour into a bowl and then add the plain Greek yoghurt, the mayonnaise, onion powder, celery salt and pepper.

Nutrition Per Serving: Calories 84; Fat 5.7g; Carbs 0.9g; Protein 10.7g; Fiber 0g; Sodium 148.5mg; Cholesterol 32.2mg

Tuna Salad

Prep Time: 10minutes

Total Time: 10 minutes

Servings: 4

Ingredients

2 tablespoons of mayonnaise

2 tablespoons of plain Greek yogurt

Juice of 1/2 lemon

2 (6-oz.) cans tuna, drained

1/4 small red onion, finely chopped

2 dill pickles, finely chopped

Freshly ground black pepper

Kosher salt

Lettuce, for serving

Directions

1. Combine the yoghurt, mayonnaise, and lemon juice in a bowl.

2. Add the drained tuna to the mayonnaise mixture. Break the tuna up into flakes. Use a fork for this.

3. Now add the red onion and then the pickles and toss to blend. Season with salt and pepper.

4. Serve on lettuce.

Vanilla Soy Pudding

Prep Time: 15 minutes

Cook Time: 5 minutes

Servings 4

Ingredients

1/4 ounce unflavored gelatin

1/4 cup of cold water

1 1/4 cup of vanilla soy milk

1 cup of tofu

1/2 teaspoon of vanilla

Directions

1. Add the cold water in a small bowl and sprinkle the gelatin over the water. Let it rest for 10 minutes to dissolve well.

2. Next, place the soy milk in a pan and heat up.

3. Add all the ingredients in a blender, including the tender gelatin and the hot soy milk and blend to smoothness. .

4. Pour into serving bowls. Chill for 2 hours.

Nutrition Per Serving: Calories 105; Fat 5g; Carbs 5g; Protein 9g; Sodium 39mg; Cholesterol 7mg

STAGE 3- Soft Foods Meal Plan

The Soft food stage is a translation to more solid foods such as soft meats, vegetables and cooked fresh fruits. Soft foods stage may last for 2 to 3 weeks. At this stage, it will easier to meet your daily protein goals without needing supplements. Men should strive to get for a daily protein intake of 60-70grams, while women should eat 50 to 60 grams. However, once you can eat between 40 -50 grams of protein in a day. reduce your intake of protein supplements.

Eat 3 meals. Add different types of low fat, starches, fruits and vegetables with low calories. Eat food in small quantities very 3 to 4 hours. Eat 5 to 6 meals each day. This is because you may not be able to eat a big meal for some months so will have to eat several small meals all through the day. Chew at least 25 times. Take chewable supplements for vitamins and minerals. Drink 48- 64 ounces of fluids, which is 6-8 cups every day.

Avoid

- Skins & seeds of fruits and vegetables
- Bread
- Raw, fibrous vegetables (broccoli and Brussels sprouts)

Suggestions For Soft Foods

Protein

- Finely ground or minced meat (chicken, turkey, beef, pork, veal)
- Finely ground seafood (tuna, whitefish shrimp or scallops)
- Bolognaise casseroles, stews and sauce
- mashed beans
- eggs

Carbs:

- Baked potatoes
- Cooked pasta with a sauce

Snacks:

- Melba toast/ breadstick/ crackers topped with humus, timmed egg, spreadable cheese

Dairy:

- Low-fat soft cheese,
- Low-fat cottage cheese

Vegetables

- Soft cooked vegetables
- Canned fruit in its own juice

SAMPLE MEAL PLAN

Breakfast

1 scrambled egg & ½ banana

Lunch

Poached fish with potatoes and broccoli

Dinner

Chicken and vegetable soup

Snacks

Grated apple

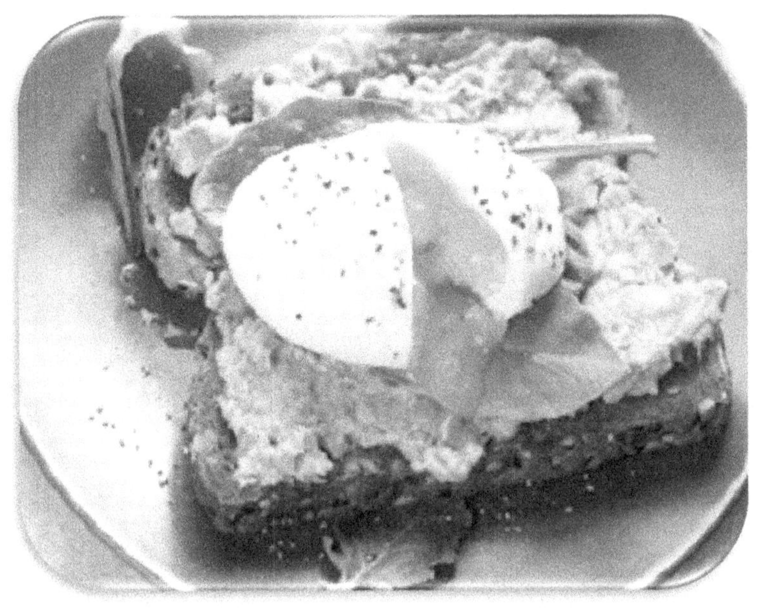

Smashed Avocado Toast With Poached Egg

A delicious protein-packed breakfast!

Prep Time: 5 minutes

Total Time: 5 minutes

Servings: 1

Ingredients

1 slice of bread, toasted

½ of 1 ripened medium avocado

Fresh lemon juice

1 hard-boiled egg

Pepper blend (Togarashi)

Extra-virgin olive oil

Kosher salt& pepper to taste

Directions

1. Smash the avocado with a fork onto the toasted slice of bread. Drizzle slightly with lemon juice.

2. Slice the egg into coins and place on the smashed avocado. Sprinkle with a little salt and pepper and an olive oil drizzle. Enjoy!

Nutrition Per Serving: Calories 309; Fat 21.2g; Carbs 22.4g; Protein 7.7g; Fiber 2g; Sodium 310.1mg;Cholesterol 186mg

Spinach & Tomato Breakfast Casserole

Another breakfast recipe packed with eggs, tomatoes, veggies& cheese. Enjoy with your family!

Prep Time: 10 minutes

Cook Time: 45 minutes

Servings: 6

Ingredients

6 eggs beaten

1/4 cup of unsalted melted butter

1/4 cup of flour

¼ cup of roasted tomatoes, chopped

½ cup of fresh spinach chopped

8 oz. small curd cottage cheese

¾ cups mozzarella cheese, shredded

1/8 teaspoon of salt

Optional Topping:

Sliced avocado

Salsa

Sour cream

Shredded Mozzarella cheese

Thinly sliced fresh chives

Directions

1. Preheat oven to 400F.

2. Spritz a baking pan with cooking spray, preferably a 9-inch x 13-inch pan.

3. Combine in a bowl; the whisked egg, melted butter the flour and the tomatoes, spinach and both cheeses. Add salt and mix well to blend. Transfer to pan.

3. Place in the oven and bake for 15 minutes. Lower temperature to 350 and bake for 30 more minutes.

4. Remove, let it cool and cut into 6 slices. Top with toppings of choice. Enjoy!

Nutrition Per Serving: Calories 232; Fat 17g; Carbs 6g; Protein 14g; Fiber 1g; Sodium 356mg; Cholesterol 202mg

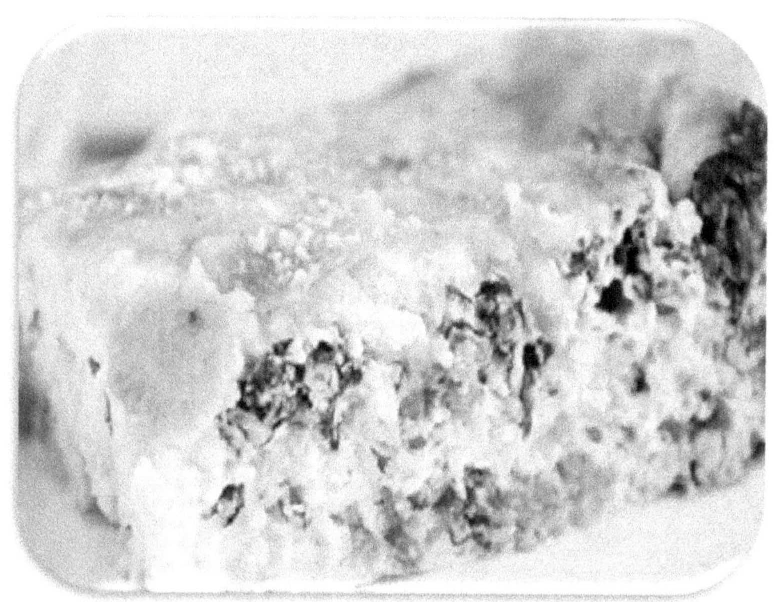

Smoked Salmon Toast

An easy breakfast option for friends to enjoy with you!

Prep Time: 10 minutes

Total Time: 10 minutes

Servings: 6

Ingredients

1 ripened avocado

1 tablespoon of crème fraîche

1 lemon

Salt and pepper, to taste

1.2 cup radishes

3 fresh dill sprigs

1 tablespoon of cider vinegar

12 slices of toasted rye bread, thinly sliced

7 ounce smoked salmon

½ pint of cress

1 handful of colorful baby leaves

Grapeseed oil

Directions

1. Halve the avocado, remove stone and scoop flesh out. Mash and add the crème fraiche and mash until very smooth. Drizzle with a little lemon juice and then add salt and pepper to season.

2. Slice the radishes finely and pick the dill and finely chop. Add the radishes and dill together in a bowl, toss with vinegar and a pinch of salt.

3. Spread the avocado over the slices of toast, top with salmon slices.

4. Sprinkle the radish slices over it, and then add the cress and leaves. Drizzle with rapeseed oil. Enjoy, served with lemon wedges.

Nutrition Per Serving: Calories 189.9; Fat 10.3g; Carbs 14g; Protein 11g; Fiber 4g;

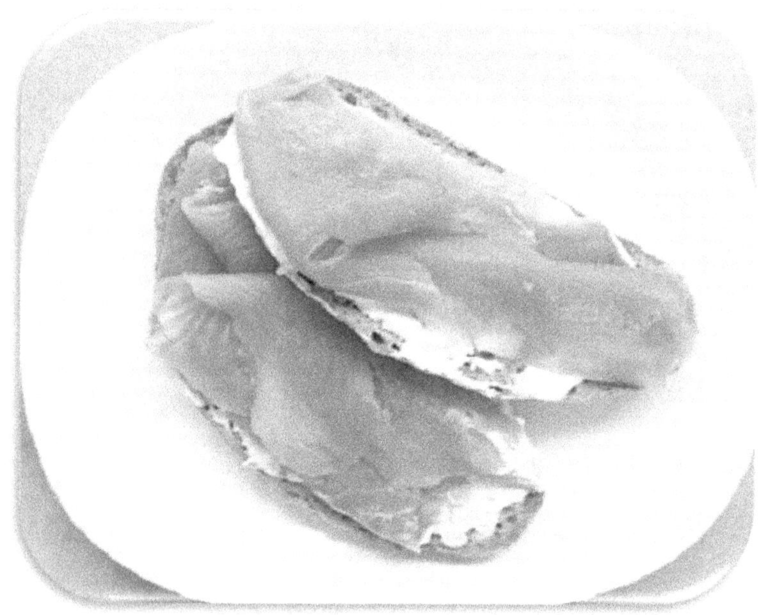

Black Bean Cakes With Guacamole

Prep Time: 10 minutes

Cook Time: 15 minutes

Servings: 4

Ingredients

1 avocado

1 tablespoon of lime juice

Salt& pepper to taste

1/4 cup of bread crumbs

1/4 cup of fresh garlic, chopped

1 teaspoon of cumin

3 teaspoons canola oil

1/4 cup tomato, chopped

1 can (15 oz.) of black beans

Directions

1. Mash the avocado in a bowl and add the lime juice as well as a little salt and pepper, stir and refrigerate.

2. Drain the canned black beans and rinse. Add to a bowl together with the breadcrumbs, cumin garlic, and oil. Mash to blend well.

3. Add oil to a pan and place over medium heat. Form bean mixture into 4 patties and add to the hot oil. Let it cook on both sides for 5 minutes until browned.

4. Serve, topped with the chilled guacamole and the chopped tomato.

Nutrition Per Serving: Calories 226.8; Fat 10.6g; Carbs 27.2g; Protein 8.1g; Fiber 8g; Sodium 164.4mg; Cholesterol 0mg

Cauliflower Soup

Prep Time: 15 minutes

Cook time: 25 minutes

Servings: 3

Ingredients:

3 bacon slices, chopped

2 cups of chicken broth

¾ cup of low fat cheese, shredded and divided

2 tablespoons of onion, chopped

½ cup sour cream

1 garlic cloves, crushed

1 green onion

1 cauliflower head, cut into florets

1 celery stalk, chopped

Salt &pepper

Directions:

1. In an instant pot, select the sauté option and cook the bacon, while frequently stirring, until it becomes crispy. Reserve the grease in the pot and transfer the bacon to a plate lined with paper towels.

2. Add the celery, onion, garlic, salt and pepper. Cook for about 4 minutes until tender. Switch off the sauté option.

3. Deglaze the pot with the broth and add the cauliflower. Cover the lid and seal the vents. Select the manual option and cook for 5 minutes at high pressure. When time us up, naturally release the pressure for 10 minutes before you open the vent.

4. Add the cream and a cup of cheese; stir and blend with an immersion blender until smooth. You can also blend in a food processor or a regular blender.

5. Add the bacon, green onion and remaining cheese as toppings.

Nutrition Per Serving: Calories 325; Fat 23.9g; Carbs 8.22g; Protein 14.7g; Fiber 2.8g;

Arugula Turkey Salad

Settle down to this tasty salad in a total of 5 minutes.

Prep Time: 5 minutes

Cook time: 0 minute

Servings: 2

Ingredients:

4 ounces of turkey breast, chopped into pieces

3.5 ounces of arugula leaves

10 berries, blueberries or raspberries

1 cucumber, peeled & then chopped

½ lime, juiced

2 tablespoons of extra virgin olive oil

Directions:

Toss all the ingredients together in a bowl.

Nutrition Per Serving: Calories 260; Fat 15g; Carbs 9g; Protein 20g; Fiber 3g;

Egg Salad

Sweet and savory!

Prep Time: 3 minutes

Cook Time: 2 minutes

Servings: 4

Ingredients:

½ cup of full fat mayonnaise

6 hardboiled eggs, peeled & chopped into pieces

1 teaspoon of curry powder

Chopped fresh parsley

Directions:

1. Combine the curry powder, eggs and mayonnaise in a bowl.

2. Serve with the parsley.

Nutrition Per Serving: Calories 305; Fat 29g; Carbs 1.7g; Protein 8.7g; Fiber 0.3g;

Creamed Spinach

Enjoyed with your favorite protein.

Prep Time: 5 minutes

Cook Time: 15 minutes

Servings: 2

Ingredients:

12 oz. fresh baby spinach

1/2 cup of heavy whipping cream

1/2 cup of grated parmesan cheese

1/4 cup of diced onion

2 garlic cloves

2 tablespoons of salted butter

Shaved parmesan cheese

Directions:

1. In a large pot, cook the spinach for about 5 minutes over medium high heat until it wilts and most of its liquid evaporated; stir constantly.

2. Turn down heat to medium and add the butter and onions; cook for about 5 minutes until the onions are soft and the butter has melted; stir constantly.

3. Stir in the Parmesan cheese until it melts.

4. Add the whipping cream and simmer over medium high heat for some minutes; stir frequently.

5. Turn down heat to low and add the garlic; stir for 1 minute until it is well mixed.

6. Taste and adjust seasoning if necessary. Garnish with shaved Parmesan and serve hot.

Nutrition Per Serving: Calories 407; Fat 39g; Carbs 8.5g; Protein 12g;

Mashed Sweet Potatoes

Prep Time: 15 minutes

Cook Time: 4 hours

Servings: 2-3

Ingredients:

1 pound of sweet potatoes, peeled & cubed

2 cloves garlic, minced

1 tablespoons of light sour cream

½ tablespoon of butter

¼ cup of 1% milk

Salt

Freshly cracked ground pepper

Directions:

1. Put the potatoes in a slow cooker and cover with water; add salt to season.

2. Cover and cook on low for 4 hours.

3. Meanwhile, melt butter in a small pan, just before the potatoes are done, and cook the garlic until it is a bit golden.

4. Use a colander to drain the potatoes and return to the slow cooker.

5. Add the sour cream, milk and sautéed garlic butter to the slow cooker; mash together until it becomes creamy and smooth.

6. Add salt and pepper to season.

Nutrition Per Serving: Calories 151; Fat 3.5g; Carbs 27g; Protein 3g;

Creamy Chicken with Squash & Apples

Prep time: 10 minutes

Cook time: 30 minutes

Servings: 4

Ingredients

8 oz. ground chicken

1/4 cup low-fat milk

1 can Cream of Chicken Soup, low-fat

1 small apple peeled, diced

½ cup of frozen butternut squash

¼ cup of shredded cheddar cheese

¼ cup whole wheat panko breadcrumbs

Directions

1. Preheat oven to 350F.

2. Add the chicken to a pan and cook. Pour in the milk and the cream of chicken soup and mix well to blend.

3. Cook over medium heat until the sauce bubbles. Now add the diced apples and then the butternut squash.

4. Transfer to a baking dish and then spread the cheese over it. Top with the panko breadcrumbs and place in the preheated oven.

5. Bake for 10 minutes.

Nutrition Per Serving: Calories 150; Fat 7g; Carbs 8g; Protein 12g; Fiber 1g; Sodium 113mg; Cholesterol 56mg

Cabbage Soup

This soup has just the right amount of kick.

Prep Time: 5 minutes

Cook Time: 20 minutes

Servings: 5

Ingredients:

(5-oz) canned diced tomatoes and green chilies

1lb. 90% lean ground beef

1 large cabbage head, chopped

1/2 teaspoon of ground cumin

2 bouillon cubes

3 cups of water

1 garlic clove, crushed

1 small onion, chopped

Salt & pepper

Directions:

1. In an instant pot, select the sauté option and brown the meat.

2. Add the onion and sauté until it is translucent.

3. Add the rest of the ingredients and stir to combine.

4. Cook for 15 minutes at high pressure using quick release.

Nutrition Per Serving: Calories 261; Fat 18g; Carbs 6g; Protein 17g; Fiber 2g;

Turkey Meatballs

Easy, soft, and undeniably delicious!

Prep time: 15 minutes

Cook time: 15 minutes

Servings: 20

Ingredients

Meatballs:

1/3 cup grated Parmesan cheese

1/3 cup whole wheat Italian-seasoned breadcrumbs

3 tablespoons fresh herbs, finely chopped

1 teaspoon kosher salt

1/2 teaspoon onion powder

1/2 teaspoon garlic powder

1/2 teaspoon dried oregano

1/4 teaspoon black pepper

1 lb. lean ground turkey

1 large egg

1 1/2 tablespoons extra-virgin olive oil

Directions

1. Preheat oven to 375F.

2. Line a rimmed baking sheet with foil, then coat it with nonstick cooking spray.

3. Add together the cheese, the whole wheat breadcrumbs, fresh herbs, salt, onion powder, garlic powder, pepper and oregano. Stir to blend all and then add the ground turkey.

4. Whisk the egg in a bowl and add to the turkey mixture. Mix gently.

5. Scoop the meat and form into 1 1/2-inch meatballs. Place on the lined and greased baking sheet and brush with olive oil.

6. Bake 15 minutes. Use an internal temperature to check that it is 165F.

7. Serve with warmed sauce.

Nutrition Per Serving: Calories 62; Fat 7g; Carbs 2g; Protein 5g; Fiber 1g; Sodium 188mg; Cholesterol 26mg

Slow Cooker Black Beans Soup
Just dump it all in your slow cooker.

Prep time: 5 minutes

Cook time: 8 hours

Servings: 4

Ingredients:

1 (110-oz) can of black beans

4 cups of boiling water

1 (24-oz) of mild chunky salsa

4 teaspoons of chicken flavored base

Directions:

1. Stir all the ingredients together in a slow cooker.

2. Cover and cook for 8 hours on low.

Nutrition Per Serving: Calories 131.6; Fat 0.6g; Carbs 23.7g; Protein 8.1g;

Homemade Vegetarian Chili

Smoky, flavorful chili of healthy vegetables and spices!

Prep Time: 20 minutes

Cook Time: 40 minutes

Servings: 2-3

Ingredients

1 tablespoon extra-virgin olive oil

1 small red onion, chopped

1 small red bell pepper, chopped

1 medium carrot, chopped

1 rib celery, chopped

¼ teaspoon salt, divided

2 garlic cloves, minced

1 tablespoon chili powder

¾ teaspoon smoked paprika

1 teaspoon ground cumin

½ teaspoon dried oregano

1small can (15 ounces) diced tomatoes, with their juices

½ can (8oz.) pinto beans, rinsed, and drained

1 can (15 ounce) black beans, rinsed, drained

1 cup vegetable broth

1 bay leaf

1tablespoon fresh cilantro, chopped

1 lime juice, to taste

Directions

1. Add olive oil to pot and heat over medium heat. Add the onions, bell pepper, the carrot, the celery and a dash of salt. Stir and cook for about 10 minutes, with occasional stirring.

2. Add the garlic, chili powder, smoked paprika, cumin and oregano to the tender vegetables in the pot and cook and stir for a minute.

3. Now add the diced tomatoes, along with their juices, the drained pinto and black beans, the broth and the bay leaf. Stir and simmer, Cook and stir every now and then for about 30 minutes.

4. Remove from heat, discard bay leaf.

5. Blend the chili for some seconds with an immersion blender. Add the chopped cilantro and mix and then add the lime juice and salt to taste

6. Divide into bowls, garnish as desired and serve.

Nutrition Per Serving: Calories 236; Fat 6.7g; Carbs 37.6g; Protein 10.9g; Fiber 10.3g; Sodium 1071mg; Cholesterol 0mg

Strawberry Cheesecake Pie

Refreshing and simple to make!

Prep Time: 10 minutes

Total Time: 10 minutes

Servings: 8

Ingredients

2 cups of sliced fresh strawberries

1/4 cup of chopped almonds, toasted

1 tablespoon of sugar

1 (9 inches) graham cracker crust

1 pkg. (8 oz.) cream cheese, softened

1 package (3.4 ounces) dry vanilla pudding mix

2 cups of cold 2% milk, divided

Directions

1. Add together in a bowl, the strawberries, the toasted almonds and the sugar. Pour mixture into crust and set aside.

2. Whisk the cream cheese in a small bowl until smooth and then add just 1/2 cup of milk. Add the instant pudding mix and the rest of the milk. Beat well and when it is well mixed, pour over the strawberries.

3. Refrigerate, covered, for at least 2 hours, to get it set.

Nutrition Per Serving (1 slice) Calories 189; Fat 6.7g; Carbs 25g; Protein 9g; Fiber 1g; Sodium 311mg; Cholesterol 3mg

Pineapple Meatballs

Prep Time: 25 minutes

Cook Time: 35minutes

Servings: 3

Ingredients

For the Meatballs:

1lb. lean ground beef

1large egg

¼ cup of fine dry breadcrumb

Dash freshly ground black pepper

½ teaspoon kosher salt

¾ teaspoons of Worcestershire sauce

Dash garlic powder

Sauce:

½ cup of packed brown sugar

11/2 tablespoons of cornstarch

3/4 cup reserved pineapple juice + water

¾ tablespoon soy sauce

1/8 cup of white vinegar

¾ teaspoon Worcestershire sauce

½ (7 ounce) can pineapple tidbits, juice drained, reserved

Directions

1. Preheat oven to 350F.

2. Add all the meatballs together in a bowl and form into balls of about 1 inches.

3. Brown and drain on paper towels and then place in a large casserole dish.

4. Make the sauce by adding together the brown sugar and the cornstarch in a large pan. Add the pineapple juice plus water and mix well until smooth.

5. Add the soy sauce, vinegar and the Worcestershire sauce. Mix together and simmer for about 5 minutes on medium-low heat. Do not cover.

6. Pour the sauce over the meatballs. Add the pineapple tidbits to it; gently stir to ensure meatballs are thoroughly coated with sauce.

7. Bake 30 minutes in the preheated oven.

Nutrition Per Serving (1 slice) Calories 559.5; Fat 17.4g; Carbs 65.3 g; Protein 34.7 g; Fiber 1.6 g; Sodium 869.4 mg; Cholesterol160.3 mg

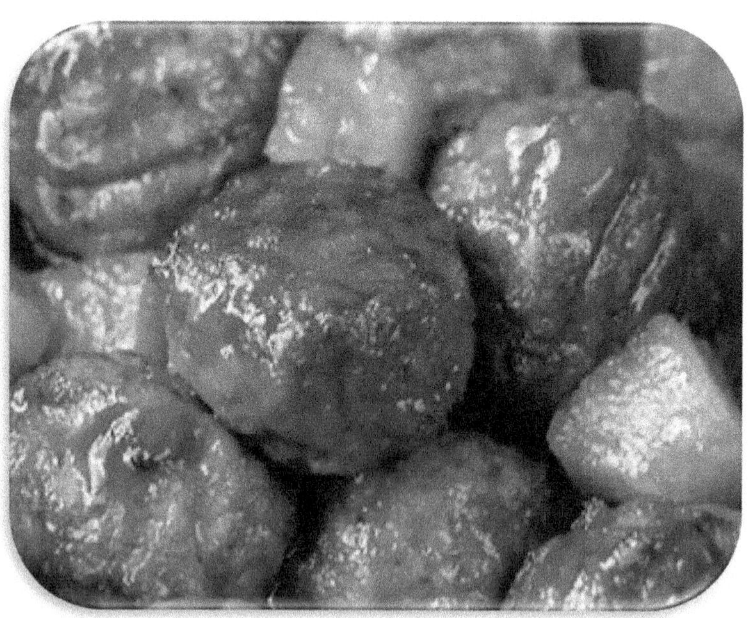

Parmesan Oven Baked Tomatoes

Ripe juicy tomatoes with an appealing garlicky parmesan crust that's well baked!

Prep Time: 5minutes

Cook Time: 10minutes

Servings: 6

Ingredients

3 large ripe tomatoes halved

¾ cup fresh bread crumbs

¼ cup freshly grated parmesan cheese

1 garlic clove minced

1 tablespoon extra-virgin olive oil

3 tablespoons of fresh herbs (basil, parsley, and oregano)

Salt& black pepper

Directions

1. Preheat oven to 400°F.

2. In a small bowl, add together the breadcrumbs, parmesan cheese, minced garlic, oil, fresh herbs, and season with salt and pepper. Toss to mix.

3. Place the sliced tomatoes in a baking dish, add a little salt & pepper. Top with the breadcrumb mixture.

4. Transfer to oven and bake for 10minutes or thereabouts.

Nutrition Per Serving Calories 53; Fat 3g; Carbs 3g; Protein 2g; Fiber 1.6 g; Sodium 72mg; Cholesterol3mg

Protein-Packed Cheesecake

Prep Time: 10 minutes

Cook Time: 1 hour

Servings: 9

Ingredients

16oz Greek yogurt cream cheese

10oz plain Greek yogurt

2 whole eggs

1/2 cup of 2% milk

2 scoops level1 protein powder

1 teaspoon vanilla extract

Salt to taste

Directions

1. Preheat oven to 300F.

2. Press cream cheese into the side of the bowl to soften. Add eggs and whisk together. Add the rest of the ingredient and blend with a mixer for 5 minutes

3. Pour into greased pan and bake for 25 minutes. Lower temperature to 180F and bake for 30 more minutes.

4. Slice in 9 pieces.

Nutrition Per Serving Calories 171; Fat 8g; Carbs 8g; Protein 17g

Spicy Coconut Mussels

Prep Time: 30 minutes

Cook Time: 10 minutes

Servings: 2

Ingredients

2 tablespoons of coconut oil

1 shallot

1 stalk lemongrass

3 garlic cloves

½ jalapeno

1 cup unsweetened coconut milk

2 pounds fresh mussels

1 teaspoon of lemon juice, or more

Zest of 1/2 lemon

½ teaspoon of Chinese fish sauce, or more

½ cup of cilantro leaves

1- 2 croissants split in half.

Directions

1. Prepare the ingredients. Finely chop the shallots and garlic clove. Trim the lemon grass, remove outer layers and chop finely. Seed the jalapeno and chop finely. Rinse the mussels.

2. Now add oil to a large pot and once hot, add the shallot, the garlic, the lemongrass and jalapeno.

3. Cover and cook about 7 minutes until the mussels have opened (discard any unopened ones).

4. Remove pot from heat, and transfer the mussels to a bowl.

5. Add the lemon zest and juice to the pot and then add fish sauce and then the cilantro. Taste and adjust seasonings as needed.

6. Meanwhile preheat the broiler. Place the croissants, on a small baking sheet. Place in the broiler for a few minutes and then remove when it's starts to become golden.

7. Put the mussels in shallow bowls. Pour over the broth and serve with the broiled croissants.

Nutrition Per Serving Calories 869; Fat 53g; Carbs 42g; Protein 60g; Fiber 2g; Sodium 1536mg;

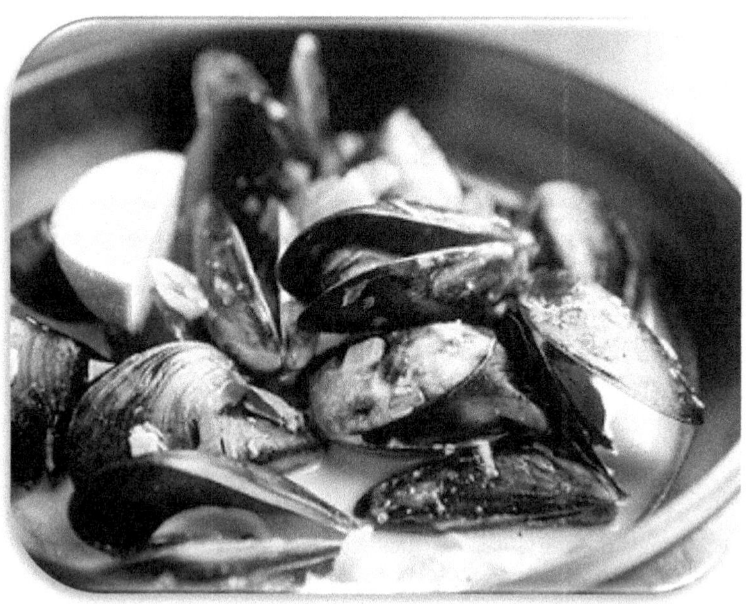

Thai Salmon and Coconut Noodles

Prep Time: 35minutes

Cook Time: 10 minutes

Servings: 4

Ingredients

12 oz. noodles

8 oz. green beans, cut into pieces of about 2 inches

1 tablespoon of canola oil

3 scallions, sliced thinly

1 small ginger, peeled, cut into matchsticks

1 jalapeño, seeded& sliced thinly

3/4 tsp. ground coriander

1/4 tsp. ground turmeric

1 15-oz. can light coconut milk

1 teaspoon of fresh lime zest

3 tablespoons of lime juice

1 1/4 lb. skinless salmon, cut into 4 pieces

1 teaspoon reduced-sodium soy sauce

1 cup of fresh cilantro leaves

Directions

1. Add water to a large pot and bring to a boil. Cook the noodles and add the green beans at the last 3 minutes of cooking. Drain noodles and rinse.

2. In the meantime, add oil to a deep skillet and heat and then add the scallions (green parts) and then add the ginger, ½ of the jalapeno and then cook and stir for a minute.

3. Add the turmeric and the coriander. Cook and stir 30 seconds. Pour in the coconut milk, ¼ cup water and the lime zest. Simmer gently and then add the salmon. Cover and cook for 5 minutes until opaque.

4. Remove from the heat and add lime juice, soy sauce, and half of the cilantro.

5. Divide the noodles, the green beans, and fish among bowls. Top with coconut broth. Sprinkle with the scallion greens, add the cilantro and the jalapeño.

Nutrition Per Serving Calories 565; Fat 9g; Carbs 69g; Protein 41g; Fiber 4g; Sodium 395mg; Cholesterol 395mg

Roasted Garlicky Brussels Salmon

Prep Time: 20 minutes

Cook Time: 25 minutes

Servings: 6

Ingredients:

2 lb. salmon fillet, wild-caught, skinned then sliced into 6 pieces

4 large garlic cloves, divided

6 cups Brussels sprouts, trimmed then sliced

¼ cup olive oil

2 tablespoons of fresh oregano, divided, finely diced

¾ cup white wine

¾ teaspoon of fresh ground pepper, divided

1 teaspoon kosher salt, divided

Lemon wedges

Directions:

1. Preheat the oven to 450°F.

2. In a small bowl, mince 2 garlic cloves with oil, ¼ tsp of pepper, 1 tbsp of oregano and ½ teaspoon of salt. Slice the remaining garlic in half; in a large roasting pan, toss the garlic with 3 tbsp of seasoned oil and Brussels. Roast for 15 minutes, stirring once.

3. Pour the wine into the remaining oil mixture then take out the pan from the oven. Stir the veggies then set the salmon on top.

4. Pour in the wine mixture slowly then sprinkle with ½ tsp of pepper, the rest of the oregano and ½ tsp of salt.

5. Bake for 5 to 10 minutes until the salmon is cooked through then serve with lemon wedges.

Nutrition Per Serving Calories 334; Fat 15g; Carbs 10g; Protein 33g; Sodium 485mg; Cholesterol 71mg

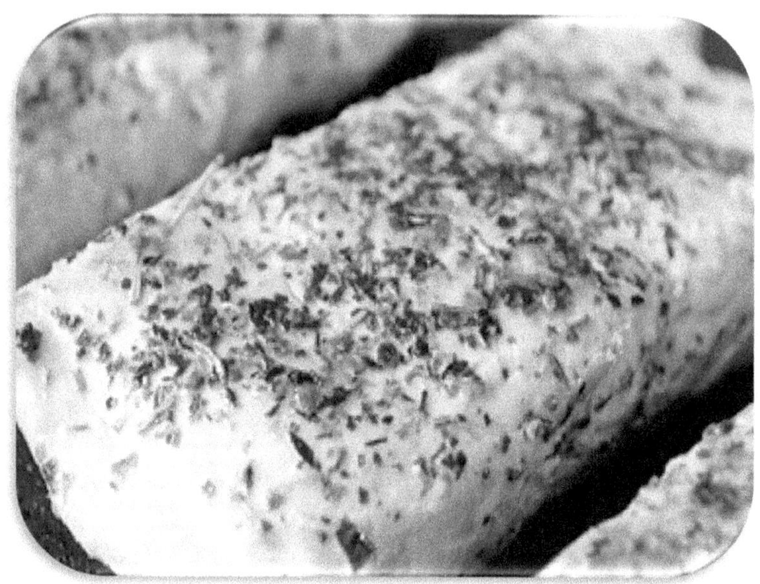

One-Pan Veggie Roasted Chicken

Enjoy a healthy dinner of roasted chicken with deliciously seasoned veggies. Yummy!

Prep Time: 5 minutes

Cook Time: 15 minutes

Servings 2

Ingredients:

2 medium chicken breasts, diced

1 cup of broccoli florets

1 cup of bell pepper, diced

1 zucchini, diced

½ onion, diced

½ cup of tomatoes, diced (or grape/plum)

¼ tsp of paprika (optional)

2 tbsp of olive oil

½ tsp of black pepper

1 tsp Italian seasoning

½ tsp salt

Directions:

1. Preheat the oven to 500°F.

2. Dice all the vegetables into chunky pieces. Chop the chicken into cubes on a separate cutting board.

3. Transfer the cubed chicken and veggies to a medium-sized sheet pan/roasting dish then add olive oil, paprika, Italian seasoning, pepper and salt, and then toss to combine.

4. Bake for about 15 minutes until the chicken is cooked and the vegetables are charred. Serve with pasta, salad or rice. Enjoy.

Nutrition Per Serving Calories 241; Fat 15.2g; Carbs 6g; Protein 19.9g; Sodium 357mg; Cholesterol 55.7mg

STAGE 4- Solid Foods Meal Plan

Good news! You've made it this far and now it's the time to start enjoying solid foods as recommended by your doctor.

However eat these foods with caution as they are difficult to digest:

- Beef & pork
- Shellfish
- Grapes
- Nuts
- whole grains
- corn
- beans

Eat in moderation:

- Small amounts of fats
- very small amounts of sugar
- Carbonated and caffeinated beverages

Totally avoid:

- Refined carbohydrate foods
- Greasy and spicy foods.

But enjoy:

- More cooked and raw fruits and vegetables
- lean meats
- Canned tuna and salmon.
- Nutrient dense foods (whole fruits, vegetables, meats, eggs).

SAMPLE MEAL PLAN

Breakfast

Baked beans on toast

Lunch

Tofu, noodles and veggie stir fry

Dinner

Baked chicken and bacon

Snacks

Chopped fruit/banana smoothie

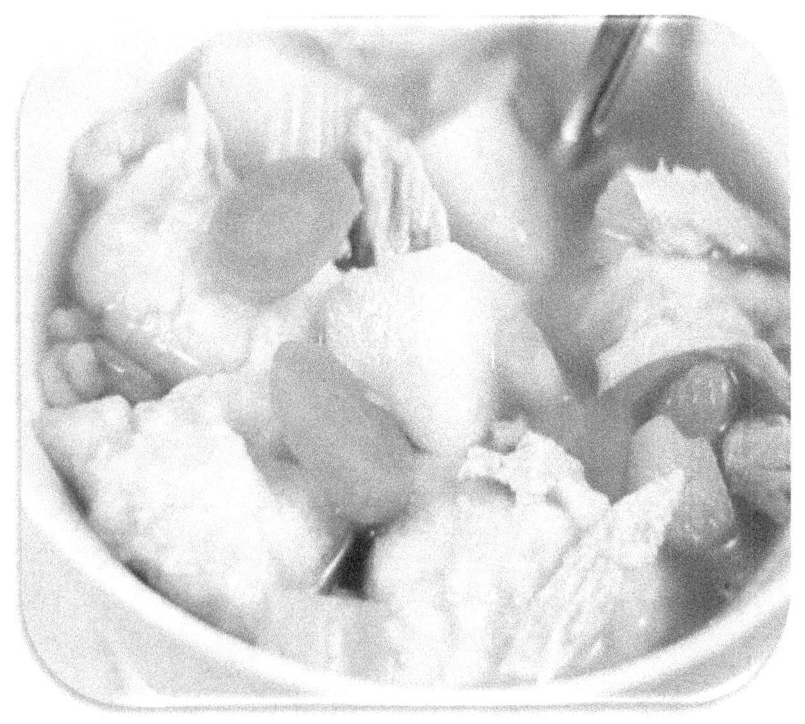

Simple Granola

The perfect base recipe for a yummy granola. Garnish and enjoy as desired.

Prep Time: 5 minutes

Cook Time: 1 hour

Servings: 16

Ingredients

1/2 cup of brown sugar

1/2 cup honey

1/4 cup vegetable oil of choice

4 cups of oats

1/2 teaspoon of cinnamon

1/4 teaspoon of salt

Directions

1. Preheat oven to 250F.

2. In a small sauce pan, add together the brown sugar, the honey and the oil and cook over medium heat. Stir to dissolve sugar and then remove.

3. Combine the oats, cinnamon and salt in a bowl and then pour over the sugar. Stir to coat the oats evenly.

4. Spread the mixture over a baking sheet, press down and bake in the oven for an hour. Stir every 15 minutes.

5. Once cooked, remove and cool. Break apart and break into pieces. Store granola in a sealed container.

Nutrition Per Serving: Calories 166; Fat 5g; Carbs 29g; Protein 3g; Fiber: 2g; Sodium 40mg

Quinoa Breakfast Bowl

Enjoy this loaded breakfast porridge.

Prep Time: 15 minutes

Cook Time: 15 minutes

Servings: 1

Ingredients

3/4 cup water, divided

1/4 cup quinoa, rinsed

2 tablespoons dried goji berries

1 small banana

1/4 cup of unsweetened almond milk

1 tablespoon of maple syrup

1/8 teaspoon of vanilla extract

1/8 teaspoon of ground cinnamon

1/4 cup of unsweetened blueberries

1 tablespoon of slivered almonds

1 tablespoon walnuts, chopped

1 tablespoon of fresh pumpkin seeds

Additional unsweetened almond milk

Directions

1. Add ½ cup water to a small saucepan and bring to a boil. Add the quinoa. Set heat to low, cover and simmer for 15 minutes to absorb liquid.

2. While it cooks, add the berries to remaining water and soak for 10 minutes, drain. Cut the banana in half crosswise. Slice I half; mash the other

3. Remove cooked quinoa from heat; fluff with a fork. Add the mashed banana to the quinoa. Add the almond milk, the maple syrup and then the vanilla and cinnamon. Mix and transfer to bowls.

4. Add the blueberries, silvered walnuts, pumpkin seeds, almonds and banana slices. Serve with additional almond.

Nutrition Per Serving: Calories 475; Fat 13g; Carbs 73g; Protein 13g; Fiber 1og; Sodium 85mg;Cholesterol 0mg

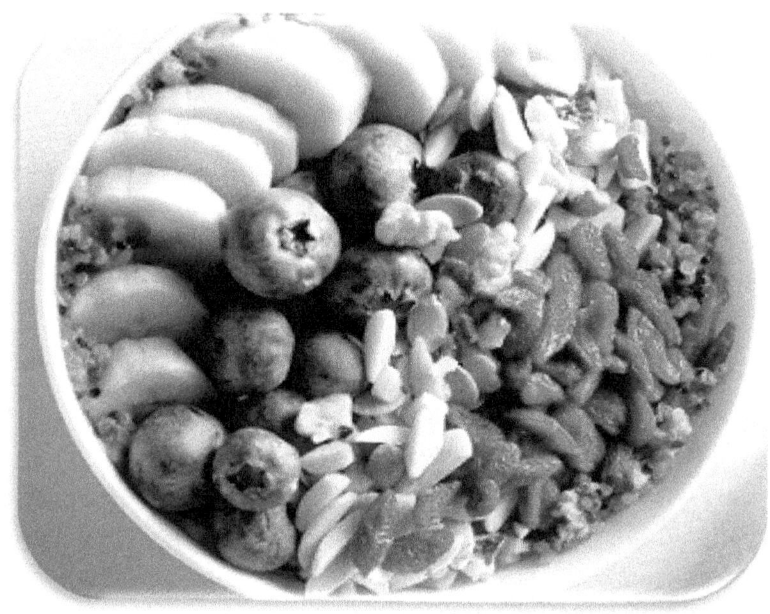

Leek And Mushroom Soup

Prep Time: 25 minutes

Cook Time: 20 minutes

Servings: 4

Ingredients:

4 cups of chicken or vegetable stock

12 medium-size Swiss brown mushrooms, sliced

2 tablespoons of olive oil or ghee

3 bay leaves

2 garlic cloves, minced

½ ounce of dried porcini mushrooms

2 medium-size potatoes, peeled and diced

1 tablespoon of dried thyme leaves

2 large-size carrots, chopped

1 leek, sliced, tough ends discarded

Pepper

Salt

Directions:

1. Put the dried mushrooms in a bowl and cover with boiling water. Leave to soak for 20 minutes.

2. Heat the olive oil over medium heat in a large pot. Add the garlic and leek, sauté until tender.

3. Add in the carrots, potatoes and thyme to the pot. Cook and stir for 2 minutes.

4. Add the rest of the ingredients and allow the soup boil. Turn down the heat to low and leave the soup to simmer until the veggies are soft.

Tomato And Basil Couscous Salad
Enjoy this lovely salad for a light lunch.

Prep Time: 10 minutes

Total Time: 20 minutes

Servings: 8

Ingredients

1-1/2 cups of water

1-1/2 cups of uncooked couscous

1/4 cup fresh basil leaves, sliced thinly

2 medium tomatoes, seeded & chopped

1/2 cup canola oil

1/4 cup of balsamic vinegar

1/2 teaspoon salt

1/4 teaspoon pepper

Directions

1. Add the water to a saucepan and bring to a boil. Add the couscous, stir and turn off heat. Let it stand, covered for cover 5 to10 minutes to enable it absorb the water. Fluff with a fork and let it cool.

2. Add the couscous to a bowl as well as the basil and tomatoes.

3. In a small bowl, combine the oil, balsamic vinegar, the salt and pepper and pour the dressing over the salad. Toss for even coating. Place in the refrigerator to chill.

Nutrition Per Serving: Calories 225; Fat 14g; Carbs 29g; Protein 5g; Fiber 2g; Sodium 155mg; Cholesterol 0mg

Seafood Chowder

Prep time: 20 minutes

Cook time: 30 minutes

Servings: 4

Ingredients

1 pound of fresh white fish, coarsely chopped

2 cups of chicken or fish stock

1 ½ cups of full fat coconut milk

1 cup of crab meat, chopped

10-12 shrimps, peeled and deveined

4 bacon slices, cooked and coarsely chopped

2 garlic cloves, minced

1 daikon radish, peeled and chopped

1 onion, chopped

2 tablespoons of coconut oil

Sea salt

Directions:

1. In a large pan, heat the oil over medium high heat and cook the shrimp for about 2-3 minutes on each side until pink. Set aside.

2. Cook the garlic and onion in the pan for 3-4 minutes; frequently stir.

3. Add the daikon and Cook for 4-5 minutes.

4. Add the white fish; cook for 2-3 minutes.

5. Stir in the stock and scrape the bottom of the pan for any bits.

6. Return the shrimp to the pan alongside the crab meat; cover and allow to simmer for 12-15 minutes.

7. Add the coconut milk and salt. Top with the bacon and serve.

Nutrition Per Serving: Calories 533; Fat 36g; Carbs 11g; Protein 44g;

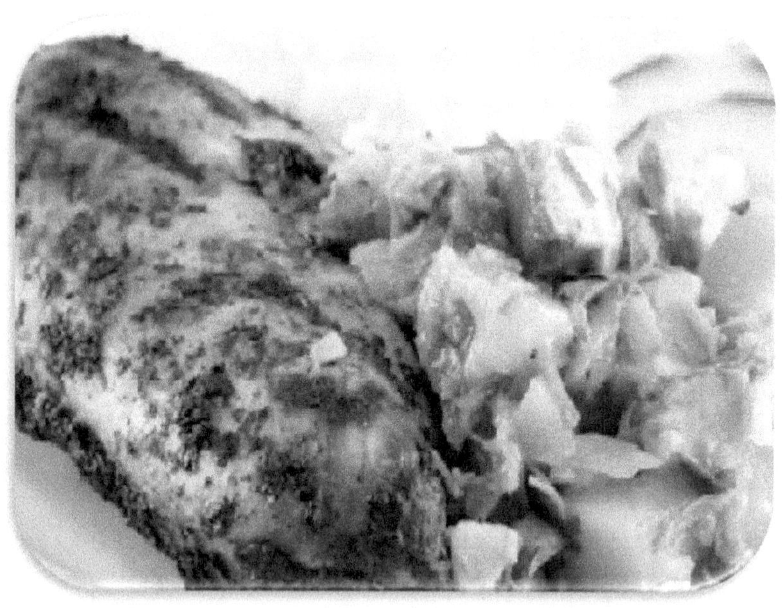

Jamaican Chicken with Mango Salsa

Jamaican Chicken with Mango Salsa

Prep Time: 15minutes

Cook Time: 10 minutes

Servings: 4

Ingredients

1/2 teaspoon Jamaican jerk seasoning

1/2 teaspoon salt, divided

4 (6-oz.) skinless, boneless chicken breast halves

Cooking spray

1/4 cup of minced fresh cilantro

1/4 cup red onion, finely chopped

1 tablespoon of chopped fresh mint

1 teaspoon of brown sugar

2 teaspoons of fresh lime juice

1/4 teaspoon crushed red pepper

1/4 teaspoon of black pepper

1 (16-oz.) jar sliced & then peeled mango, drained & chopped

Directions

1. Season the chicken with ¼ teaspoon of salt and the jerk seasoning. Spritz with cooking spray

2. Brown the chicken in a large pan on both sides for 10 minutes.

3. Add together the remaining salt, the cilantro and the rest of the ingredients.

4. Enjoy the cooked chicken with the salsa.

Nutrition Per Serving: Calories 224; Fat 2.4g; Carbs 14.7g; Protein 39.8g; Fiber 1.6g; Sodium 445mg; Cholesterol 99mg

Chicken Cordon Bleu

Prep Time: 15 minutes

Cook Time: 30 minutes

Servings: 4

Ingredients

8 ham, thinly sliced

8 oz. Swiss cheeses sliced

4 (2 lb.) boneless skinless chicken breasts,

Salt and pepper

3 cups panko breadcrumbs

6 tablespoons melted butter

Sauce:

1 cup of mayonnaise

1-2 teaspoons yellow mustard

Directions

1. Pat dry chicken with paper towel, cut in half to create 2 halves of chicken breast.

2. Place chicken between plastic wrap sheets and pound thinly and evenly with a meat mallet

3. Top chicken pieces with a ham slice and shredded cheese and then roll and tuck the sides gently. Cover with another sheet of plastic wrap, wrap chicken tightly and twisting to make the roll firm.

4. Chill 45 minutes to 24 hours.

5. Preheat oven to 400F. Unwrap chicken, season with salt and pepper. Dip in melted butter and coat in breadcrumbs. Grease baking sheet lightly and then place the chicken on it.

6. Bake 30 minutes, or more.

7. Combine the mustard and mayo and enjoy with the chicken.

Nutrition Per Serving: Calories 657; Fat 35g; Carbs 19g; Protein 63g; Sodium 445mg; Cholesterol 232mg

Vegetable Soup

Prep time: 15 minutes

Cook time: 20 minutes

Servings: 6

Ingredients

8 cups of reduced sodium vegetable or chicken broth

6 cups of chopped vegetables

Salt

Directions:

1. Simmer the vegetables and broth in a large pot over high heat; lower heat, partially uncover the pot and simmer until the veggies are soft.

2. Blend the soup until smooth with a regular or immersion blender and season with salt.

Nutrition Per Serving: Calories 272; Fat 8g; Carbs 44g; Protein 8g;

Baked Eggplant Parmesan

A delicious classic Italian for the whole family will love!

Prep Time: 30 minutes

Cook Time: 25 minutes

Servings: 6

Ingredients

<u>Basic Sauce</u>

1 can (14oz.) peeled tomatoes

2 tablespoons extra virgin olive oil

2 garlic cloves, minced

1/4 teaspoon of kosher salt

1/2 teaspoon of oregano

5 leaves fresh basil, chopped

1/4 cup of water

<u>Layers</u>

3 medium Italian eggplants, sliced about ¼ inches

1 1/2 cups of firm mozzarella shredded

3/4 cup of Parmesan cheese

Directions

1. Pre-heat oven to 350°F.

2. Place the sliced eggplant in a bowl, sprinkle with salt and let it rest for 20 minutes. Drain afterwards (don't rinse).

3. Add water to a medium pot and then add the olive oil, tomatoes, minced garlic, the oregano, salt and basil leaves. Stir and squash the tomatoes a little. Let it simmer to thicken and enable most of the water evaporate.

4. Now grill the rested eggplant.

5. Spread a little sauce on a baking dish of about 8 by 6 inches. Add the grilled eggplant, top with sauce and then the mozzarella cheese and the Parmesan and finally top the last layer with parmesan cheese. This should make 3-4 layers. Place the dish on a cookie sheet.

6. Transfer to oven and bake 30 minutes. Cool for 5 minutes and then serve.

Nutrition Per Serving: Calories 225; Fat 15g; Carbs 13g; Protein 13g; Fiber 5g; Sodium 574mg; Cholesterol 31mg

Orange And Chicken Salad

Prep Time: 10 minutes

Cooking Time: 0 minute

Servings: 4

Ingredients:

¼ cup of lemon juice, freshly squeezed

4 handfuls of lettuce

2 tablespoons of olive oil

2 large ripe tomatoes, diced

2 oranges, peeled and sliced

2 celery stalks, sliced

1 Lebanese cucumber, diced

Meat from 1 cooked chicken

¼ cup of black olives, optional

Directions:

1. In a large bowl, put all the ingredients except the oil and lemon juice.

2. Drizzle the oil and lemon juice over it and toss to combine. Enjoy with grilled chicken.

Baked Zucchini Fries

Ultra cheesy and so flavorful!

Prep Time: 15 minutes

Cook Time: 30 minutes

Servings: 4

Ingredients

2 zucchini

1 whole egg

1 cup of Romano cheese, grated

1 teaspoon of Italian spice

1 teaspoon of garlic powder

Lemon Parsley Aioli

1/2 cup mayo

1 lemon, juiced

1 clove garlic, minced

1 tablespoon of parsley, finely chopped

Salt and pepper

Directions

1. Preheat the oven to 425F. Line 2 baking trays with parchment paper. Slice each zucchini into 16 slices. To do this, slice in half twice and then into quarters. Whisk eggs slightly in a bowl.

2. Combine the Romano cheese and spices in a separate bowl and mix to blend.

3. Dip a zucchini slice in the egg and then to the cheese mix, coating thoroughly. Place in the lined baking tray.

4. Once all zucchini are well-coated, place in the oven and bake for 30 minutes. Half way through cooking, flip. Once cooked, remove and serve.

5. Combine all the aioli ingredients together, stirring well.

6. Enjoy zucchini fried dipped in aioli.

Nutrition Per Serving: Calories 156.8; Fat 9.8g; Carbs 6.2g; Protein 12.5g; Fiber 1.6g; Sodium 258mg; Cholesterol 66mg

Spinach Dip

Prep Time: 5 minutes

Total Time: 5 minutes

Servings: 16

Ingredients

1 pkg. (10 oz.) frozen chopped spinach

1 cup mayonnaise

2 cups Greek yogurt

1 pkg. (1.4 oz.) dry vegetable soup mix

8 oz. water chestnuts canned & drained

3 green onions chopped

Directions

1. Place the spinach in fridge overnight to defrost. Squeeze dry.

2. Chop the water chestnuts.

3. Add all the ingredients together in a bowl and mix thoroughly. Place in the refrigerator for 2 hours before serving.

4. Serve with bread or crackers.

Nutrition Per Serving: Calories 174; Fat 16g; Carbs 5g; Protein 1g; Fiber 1.6g; Sodium 412mg; Cholesterol 20mg

Ginger Spiced Chicken

Prep Time: 5 minutes

Cook Time: 40 minutes

Servings: 4

Ingredients:

1½ pounds of chicken drumsticks

1 tablespoon of olive oil or ghee

1 small brown onion, chopped

1 inch of sliced fresh ginger, peeled and chopped finely

½ red pepper, sliced

½ teaspoon of salt

½ teaspoon of cayenne pepper

Directions:

1. In a pan over medium heat, put the oil.

2. Sauté the onion and garlic for 3 minutes.

3. Add the rest of the ingredients except the chicken.

4. Add the chicken, combine and reduce the heat to simmer gently.

5. Cook for 30 minutes or until the chicken is well-cooked. Stir occasionally

Spiced Lime Shrimp Salad

This salad is packed with seafood rich in Omega-3, which increases focus, mental agility and sharpness.

Prep Time: 10 minutes

Cook Time: 33 minutes

Servings: 2

Ingredients:

8 oz large shrimp, peeled, vein removed then rinsed

1½ tbsp freshly squeezed lime juice

1 tbsp chopped cilantro

1 small scallion, green and white parts, chopped

½ tsp extra-virgin olive oil

½ tbsp hoisin sauce

¼ tsp minced garlic

Pinch of ground white pepper

Bibb lettuce leaves

1 tbsp diced red bell pepper

Directions:

1. In a large bowl, combine lime juice, scallion, cilantro, oil, hoisin sauce, white pepper and garlic then whisk everything together to mix. Set aside.

2. Heat 1 tbsp of the reserved lime juice mixture in a large nonstick skillet over medium heat.

3. Add the shrimp then cook for 2 to 3 minutes, tossing until the shrimp becomes opaque.

4. Pour the contents in the skillet into the reserved lime juice mixture. Add the bell pepper, cover then refrigerate for 30 minutes, tossing from time to time.

5. Refrigerate two serving dishes if you like.

6. Line each refrigerated plate with the lettuce leaves then scoop the shrimp and some of the marinade into the lettuce.

Nutrition Per Serving: Calories 151; Fat 3.4g; Carbs 5g; Protein 24g;

CONCLUSION

Having lost up to 50- 70 % weight with your successful gastric surgery, you have to ensure you keep the weight off. Following your surgeon's diet guidelines, regular weekly exercises and eating nutrient-packed non-processed foods will do this for you.

All the best!